Culture and mental health:
a southern African view

Leslie Swartz

OXFORD UNIVERSITY PRESS

Cape Town

1998

Oxford University Press

Great Clarendon Street, Oxford OX2 6DP, United Kingdom

offices in
Oxford, New York
Athens, Bangkok, Calcutta, Cape Town, Chennai, Dar es Salaam, Delhi
Florence, Hong Kong, Istanbul, Karachi, Kuala Lumpur, Madrid, Melbourne
Mexico City, Mumbai, Nairobi, Paris, Singapore, Taipei, Tokyo, Toronto

and associated companies in
Berlin, Ibadan

Oxford is a trade mark of Oxford University Press

Culture and mental health:
a southern African view

ISBN 0 19 570981 0

COPY EDITOR: Helen Karlsen
TEXT DESIGNER: Mark Standley
INDEXER: Ethné Clarke
COVER DESIGNER: Peter Burgess

Published by Oxford University Press Southern Africa
PO Box 12119, N1 City, 7463, Cape Town, South Africa

Set in Dante by RHT desktop publishing cc, Durbanville
Printed and bound by Creda Communications
Eliot Avenue, Eppindust II, Cape Town

for Louise, Alison, and Rebecca

contents

foreword

THIRTY YEARS AGO, when I entered the field of culture and mental health, one had to first make a case for the relevance of culture. That point could not be taken for granted. Today, for several reasons, including substantial change both in the climate of the times as well as in the mental health professions themselves, the situation is entirely different. Multicultural realities are commonplace, and understood to be consequential. Globalization has projected the special practices and peculiar meanings of local worlds into lay and professional discourse world-wide to such an extent that international readers and TV audiences are prepared to encounter even the most extreme differences. It has also infiltrated virtually all local worlds via the media and face-to-face communication so that there can hardly be a local world that can any longer remain uninfluenced either by the diversity of human conditions or by the universalizing discourses (on human nature, ethics, and human rights but also about free markets and international styles).

In such a world, the emergence – or enhancement – of cultural psychology, cultural psychiatry, and psychiatric anthropology is hardly surprising. Hybrid disciplines like these play a crucial role of bridging domains that may once have seemed distant but that now are all too frequently brought into interaction. The result of this historic change also includes the publication of strong books that present the key concepts and findings of these fields. Mental health is especially well served by Leslie Swartz's volume. Here is an author who is expert in mental health yet also has read widely and deeply in anthropology and cultural studies. And he is experienced over the long haul in assessing and caring for patients from the multiplex of South African backgrounds. He brings to bear on his subject a persistently cultural focus that is especially of value because it is as able to draw on the most prominent examples from the international scholarly literature as from materials local to South Africa, where Swartz is a leading clinician-teacher.

I am as impressed by Swartz's handling of the thorny and controversial questions that so regularly lurk in the interface between cultural orientations and mental health approaches as I am by the clarity of his presentation of basic ideas and practices in psychology and psychiatry. The South African experience is obviously relevant to understanding racism, trauma, and the postmodern pluralism of healing approaches. But Swartz is also a fine guide to such standard issues as culture and depression, somatization, and the social course of chronic mental illness. He explains why the well-tried concept of culture-bound syndromes is in trouble, and what is wrong (as well as right) with the notion of posttraumatic stress disorder.

The book is also highly accessible for beginning students in psychology, nursing, social work, and even medicine. There is a judicious review of complex issues in almost every chapter. And yet Swartz doesn't avoid coming down on one side or the other. Best of all is the process of reasoning the book exhibits. Swartz draws on a great deal of published work – the breadth of the bibliography is impressive – and shows how different authors coming from divergent orientations think through the connection between cultural processes and mental health experiences in ways that demonstrate those differences. Yet, difference does not mean 'beyond understanding'. Swartz's prose comes alive in showing how differences in symptoms, life history, ethnicity, class, and gender can be understood and then applied to provide better care.

Why should the senior clinician spend his limited free time to write such a book? Since Swartz is modest in claiming originality (he credits many scholars), recognition of his own achievement will come from the record of how successful he is in getting teachers to use this book as a course text and in interesting students to pore over the text and perhaps go behind it to read some of the key articles and books listed in the bibliography. This is a labour of love that stands for Leslie Swartz's commitment to students. In making South African materials a major source of illustration, he assures that his contribution is to

South Africa as much as anywhere.

This is a rough time in South Africa. Neither blacks nor whites seem at all satisfied with the first several years of outcome of their peaceful revolution. The transfer of wealth and status from the latter to the former has not happened. Crime has increased to such a daunting degree that it has threatened the society as a whole. Perhaps a book on culture and mental health can assist a new generation of students in South Africa to become excited by this subject, and in future to address inequality, structural discrimination, and their relation to cultural difference. This book does not have that as an explicit political programme, but anyone who reads it through attentively will draw the logical conclusion. For what is at stake in this book is no more and no less than the question of how to rebuild psychology (and the other mental health fields) for a vastly different society, era, and world. In future perhaps the issue will be put this way: we are all multicultural-ists now, as Nathan Glazer puts it, and a text on culture and mental health is as basic to mental health as any other mental health textbook. Or alternatively, the world in its glorious and frustrating diversities is too immense to give itself up to unified codification by a single system. It isn't a system that we want anyway, but a method, and such a method must at heart enable a reckoning with cultural meanings and social inequalities. Eyes are on South Africa for evidence of new polit-ical and cultural transitions. It is to be hoped that Swartz's book will contribute in its own way to that very necessary (and potentially glo-bally consequential) transformation. Why shouldn't South Africa become a model of putting cultural psychology (and psychiatry) into practical programmes?

Arthur Kleinman
Chair, Department of Social Medicine
Harvard Medical School

acknowledgements

THIS BOOK OWES a great deal to many people.

Many of the ideas presented here were developed over some years in discussion with my teachers and supervisors, with colleagues, and with students. In particular I should like to thank Julia Binedell, Athalie Crawford, Andy Dawes, Gerard Drennan, Peter du Preez, Don Foster, Louise Frenkel, Kerry Gibson, Marion Holdsworth, Sharon Kleintjes, Ann Levett, Anastasia Maw, Tracey Miller, Nomsa Ngqakayi, John Reynolds, Pippa Rogers, Sharon Rumble, Monica Spiro, Sally Swartz, and Hester van der Walt.

The staff of the Child Guidance Clinic at the University of Cape Town provided support and help in many ways, and the Inter-Library Loans Department of the Jagger Library at the University of Cape Town were consistently helpful. Sabbatical leave granted by the University of Cape Town gave me the time to write the book.

Drafts were read and helpfully commented on by Bev Dickman, Louise Frenkel, Gerard Drennan, Kerry Gibson, Anastasia Maw, and Valerie Sinason. Louise Frenkel provided much-needed emotional support and sustenance. Thanks also to Alison and Rebecca Swartz.

Without the stories of many clients and research respondents, this book would not have been possible.

Oxford University Press commissioned the book, and I should like to thank the staff of Oxford University Press and their freelance editors.

Financial support for parts of this work was provided by the Centre for Science Development. Community projects financed by Rädda Barnen (Swedish Save the Children) provided me with many learning opportunities in the field of culture and mental health.

In spite of all the help I have received, I must take full responsibility for this work. The opinions I express are mine and are those of no other person or organization.

PART I

Looking at culture and
mental health and illness

I

Ways of seeing

What is the relationship between culture and
  mental health?
Is mental illness universal?
Are there ways of dealing with mental health
  problems which differ from culture to culture?
Do some systems work better than others?
If we had a different social order, could we reduce
  the rates of mental illness?
Is modern living bad for our mental health?

QUESTIONS OF THIS SORT ARE FASCINATING – they are asked all
the time, by all kinds of people. But it can be confusing trying to sort
out the best ways of answering them.

Claims are made in the media for great advances in the scientific
treatment of mental illness. Developments in biological sciences and
genetics hold out the eventual promise of eradicating, or at least limiting, debilitating mental illnesses such as schizophrenia. At the same
time, though, throughout the world there is increasing interest in
forms of healing which are not part of the Western medical system
(known as biomedicine). Internationally, tarot cards, crystals, wilder-
ness experiences, and 'primitive' healing rituals are gaining increasing
attention – the 'new age' business is booming. In South Africa, where
a difficult political transformation has been achieved, interest in

indigenous healing practices is probably higher than ever. There are calls for an integrated health service which draws on the strengths of biomedicine and those of indigenous healing.

What is happening to our thinking when, on the one hand, we value the contributions of laboratory science to healing, and are sceptical about all other forms of knowledge and, on the other, we claim that indigenous healing touches people and communities in a way which Western scientific medicine cannot? Things get more complicated when we also have to consider the claims made loudly against different systems of understanding and treating mental illness. Western psychiatry is accused of being conservative, of oppressing people, of forcing them against their will to conform to social roles they may not wish to take on. From another perspective, indigenous healing methods are seen by some as mumbo-jumbo, unproven in efficacy and unhelpful. Both systems of healing are seen as ways that practitioners have developed to make money. Some people say the best wisdom about keeping mentally healthy comes from generations of the experience of ordinary people, and not from professionals. Communities, we are told, know how to look after themselves, and it is the wisdom of common sense that we should take most seriously. People should be encouraged to take care of their own mental health in their own ways. Health clubs, gyms, aromatherapists, stress management practitioners all promise mental health benefits from their practices, and all emphasize the value of taking care of ourselves and taking control of our lives. Where mental health becomes a personal responsibility, however, it can become easier to blame those who are not mentally healthy. Throughout the ages, mentally ill people in all societies have been, to varying degrees, stigmatized, isolated, and open to abuse. If mental illness is seen as a consequence of being neglectful about mental health, then patterns of stigma and abuse may be reinforced.

How do we find our way through this maze of differing opinions? How do we know what to think, what to recommend when trying to improve the mental health of a diverse but increasingly interconnected world? There is no single or easy answer to these questions, and this book does not attempt to provide an answer. What this book will do, though, is provide you with some tools with which to do your own thinking about questions of culture and mental health. One approach to dealing with the topic of this book could be to give many examples of different ways people experience mental illness in different cultures, and different ways mental illness is managed. We shall indeed be learning about some of these, but the aim of this book is not to give a guided tour of mental illness around the world. This is a book about ways of seeing mental health, mental illness, and healing.

This may seem strange. Why have a book about culture and mental health which focuses not on different cultures but rather on the ways we look at different cultures? Whom are we studying? The people in the different cultures or ourselves as observers? The reason I focus on ways of looking at culture is that every question we ask about culture and mental health depends on how we see the world. Ask questions from one perspective, and you will get particular answers. Ask from another, and different answers will emerge. As we will see in this book, many of the questions which opened this chapter are just too broad to be answered simply, and depend on assumptions held by the questioners. It is our job, in trying to understand culture and mental health, to remember that no human activity is free from cultural influence. We cannot observe cultural practices without remembering that our act of observation is a cultural practice in itself.

All this leads us to the central question of how we define the terms we are using. Our first step is to think about these terms and to have a sense of what we mean about culture and mental health.

Thinking about culture

The concept of culture has occupied the minds of anthropologists and other social scientists for generations, and continues to do so. Many books have been written about culture and culture theory. As a starting point, let's consider a dictionary definition. *Webster's new twentieth century dictionary*, Second Edition (1978), provides eight different definitions of the word 'culture'. In brief, these are:

i) the act of tilling the soil for crops; *ii)* the raising or improvement of a plant or animal product; *iii)* the growth of bacteria; *iv)* a colony of bacteria grown; *v)* improvement or refinement by study or training; *vi)* the training or refining of the mind, emotions, manners, or taste; *vii)* the result of this training – refinement of thought, emotion, manners, and taste; and *viii) the concepts, habits, skills, art, instruments, institutions, etc. of a given people in a given period; civilization.*

The last of the eight definitions (which I have given in full and which I have put in italics) is clearly the one with which we will be most interested in this book, but two features of the previous definitions are important for us to note. First, the concept of culture is often concerned with growth and change. Second, some definitions of culture are concerned with a value judgement concerning refinement or sophistication – people who are sophisticated are seen as more 'cultured' than others, for example. There is a problem with using this definition of culture in the context of this book. It implies a judgement about people and the value of what they do, and it also allows for a split in how we refer to people and culture. For example, it could be said that sophisticated people go to the theatre, ballet, or opera to get their dose of culture, but that unsophisticated people live in different cultures all the time. In this view, culture (in the sense of definition viii) is something which only other people, or unsophisticated people, have. This is not the case. As we will see in this book, even the most sophisticated scientific practices operate from a cultural base.

Helman (1994) views culture as a

set of guidelines (both explicit and implicit) which individuals inherit as members of a particular society, and which tells them how to *view* the world, how to experience it emotionally, and how to *behave* in it in relation to other people, to supernatural forces or gods, and to the natural environment. It also provides them with a way of transmitting these guidelines to the next generation – by the use of symbols, language, art and ritual. (Helman, 1994: 2–3, emphasis in the original)

Culture, then, is about the process of being and becoming a social being, about the rules of a society and the ways in which these are enacted, experienced, and transmitted. Culture cannot be static, as interpretations of rules change over time with different circumstances. Many political movements in the world concern themselves with what they term 'the preservation of culture' – such as the preservation of Afrikaner culture, or the preservation of Zulu or Irish culture. Invariably, though, such movements are not about preserving something as one would preserve a laboratory specimen in formalin, but about trying to implement and/or maintain a set of power relationships in a contemporary context. It is also not possible to draw tight boundaries around cultures as though they were separate entities. We are all influenced by a variety of forces, ranging from our immediate kin group through schools, health care systems, political systems, the mass media, and, increasingly, the Internet. The image of the anthropologist going out to view strange, exotic cultures never before in contact with Western or other cultures is seriously outdated in the context of our interconnected global world.

Modern developments in the way we think about culture, though, suggest this image is problematic not only because the world is changing. Clifford (1986) has raised questions about the ways in which anthropologists have portrayed themselves as relatively passive and objective viewers of other cultures. In considering the anthropologist putting up a tent in a village being studied, Clifford points out that the anthropologist is also on view. He argues that the process of studying culture is in itself an activity with its own rules, and which needs to be problematized not simply as gathering information from exotic people. The emerging discipline of cultural psychology well amplifies the dynamic way in which culture can be viewed:

> Cultural psychology is the study of the way cultural traditions and social practices regulate, express, transform, and permute the human psyche ... Cultural psychology is the study of the ways subject and object, self and other, psyche and culture, person and context, figure and ground, practitioner and practice

live together, require each other, and dynamically, dialectically, and jointly make each other up. (Shweder, 1990: 1)

In thinking about culture, then, we are thinking as much about ourselves as about other people, as much about what we already know as about what we are finding out. We are engaged in a process not only of discovering meaning but also about making meaning.

We shall be returning to some of these issues later in this chapter and throughout this book. For now, though, it is enough to have noted some of the questions we raise when we use the word 'culture' and when we try to think about culture and mental health.

Thinking about mental health

People often have less difficulty with the concept of mental health than with the concept of culture, but the term is no less culturally loaded. White (1982: 85) asks 'What is "mental" about "mental health"?' In asking this White is referring implicitly to the kinds of categories we tend to use in dominant Western biomedical culture – and specifically to the split between body and mind. This split has a long history going back to Descartes in the seventeenth century. Western medicine is based on the idea that there are some afflictions which are purely physical in nature and others which are psychological – on the idea that it is possible to conceive of mental and physical states as separate. This view is becoming increasingly untenable, even within biomedicine, as biomedicine becomes more sophisticated both biomedically and in terms of its understanding of the social sciences (Eisenberg, 1986), but it still plays an important role in the way biomedicine divides up its areas of speciality and, specifically, in what it sees as 'mental'.

If we are going to think about culture and mental health, we need to bear in mind that the conceptual barrier biomedicine places between mental and physical health is not one which applies to all systems of thought. It does not make sense to everyone to separate the physical from the mental, and many forms of healing do not make this rigid distinction. Later in this book we will be considering the concept of somatization, which will demonstrate the difficulties people who do not share biomedicine's view of the mind/body split may face when they are treated within a biomedical system. Within biomedicine itself, the mind/body split has provided a view of the body as a machine, which has been central to many of its remarkable successes. This very split, however, is now presenting difficulties as we attempt to come to terms with increasing rates of chronic and lifestyle-related disorders. If we know, for example, that susceptibility to heart attacks may be influenced by psychological and social stressors, as we do, then do we properly consider heart attacks as mental health problems? Clearly, heart attacks have to do with the capacity of the heart as a mechanical pump, but we now know that psychological factors can play a part in whether this pump will continue to work.

This discussion leads us to the question of where we draw the boundaries around the concept of mental health. Some would say that mental health issues relate only to questions regarding disorders which are narrowly psychiatric – for example, disorders which appear in the DSM-IV (*Diagnostic and statistical manual of mental disorders* – Fourth Edition; American Psychiatric Association, 1994), a diagnostic system which will be discussed in more detail in Chapter 3. Another view, though, is expressed in the recent *World mental health* report (Desjarlais et al., 1995). This volume demonstrates the health and social impacts of a variety of problems, including violence, poverty, substance abuse, dislocation, and women's oppression in low-income countries. The authors show that the expertise of mental health practitioners can make an important impact not only on mental illnesses as narrowly defined but also on illness and mortality more generally, on the way societies work, and on the functioning of economies. The reports calls on us to take seriously the view that what mental health workers may have to offer society may be based not on their expertise with a specific range of problems or people, but a way of looking at, and contributing to, solutions for a very broad range of health and social issues. The challenges of the AIDS epidemic reinforce the view that it is a mistake to define mental health too narrowly. At present, AIDS is incurable, and the only way we can contain the epidemic is by affecting people's behaviour – largely, their sexual behaviour. Social scientists and mental health practitioners are at the forefront of this work.

This expansion in our understanding of what the 'mental' part of mental health is also relates to a consideration of what 'health' may be. In 1978, the World Health Organization proposed a view of 'health' as not merely the absence of disease or infirmity, but a positive state of physical, mental, and social well-being. In this view, mental well-being is part of health and cannot be separated from it. It is, of course, very difficult to know what mental well-being is, and the definition will differ from person to person and from context to context. It is also difficult to know when a difficulty or problem becomes a sign of mental ill-health or illness. The very terms 'health' and 'illness' locate problems in living in a medical realm, but this medicalized way of looking at problems is not common to everyone. To members of some religious groups, for example, what a psychologist might consider a mental heath problem could be viewed primarily as a spiritual problem. Other people see the world more in terms of moral issues, and so on. A central point of this book is that it is a cultural construction that we consider mental health as a health issue. The consequences of this construction are profound – for example, vast numbers of mental health problems are confronted by primary health care practitioners such as nurses, doctors, and community health workers. This is how things are. But part of our job in thinking about culture and mental health is to realize that what we might term mental health problems may be seen and dealt with in a wide variety of settings – not all of which are labelled health settings. Even hairdressers and bartenders can help to manage the mental health problems of some of their clients.

Having established, then, that the area of culture and mental health may be broader than may at first appear, let us now go on to consider some of the major theoretical approaches for dealing with the field. Understanding these will help us evaluate the material presented in subsequent chapters.

Approaches to understanding culture and mental health

What is our job in trying to understand culture and mental health? Are we trying to find out more about people's experiences? Are we wanting to describe different healing systems? Do we want to improve biomedical care in the context of a diverse patient population? Do we want to advocate a neglected or new form of alternative health care? Do we want to know how to keep ourselves and our communities mentally healthy?

All of these are legitimate aims, and to some extent they may overlap. But depending on who you are and what interests you, it is possible to adopt very different ways of thinking about culture and mental health. For example, some people who write in this area are psychiatrists who are convinced that biological causes and treatments will be found for the majority of serious emotional disorders. Others are traditional healers who feel that their own perspective on mental health has been largely ignored in the literature. Still others are social scientists wishing to expose financial interests behind certain forms of research and intervention. Throughout this book it will be important to bear in mind that there is a range of views and that all views, however well expressed (including my own), must relate to some degree to the interests of those expressing them. What follows in this chapter, therefore, is not simply a summary of three major approaches but a consideration of why these approaches are attractive and to whom. In practice, few authors keep strictly to one approach, and many move around across approaches. There are also many ways of categorizing different approaches (Carter & Qureshi, 1995; Kleinman, 1977; Scheper Hughes & Lock, 1987). For ease of presentation, I shall first identify universalist approaches to the field, then relativism, and finally critical approaches.

1 Universalism

Introducing his book on transcultural psychiatry, Leff (1988) tells the story of two butterfly collectors, one in Britain and the other in

Nigeria. The British collector has discovered a butterfly he calls the 'Battersea Beauty', and the Nigerian a butterfly he calls the 'Ibadan Imperial'. Through a process of correspondence they find that, although they have been using different words to describe the butterflies, the collectors have found examples of the same butterfly – they have been talking about the same thing.

This tale well summarizes the central project of universalist approaches to understanding mental health and illness. The fundamental assumption of universalism is that mental illness is universal, and that our job in looking cross-culturally is to find evidence for these universals. Two things may obscure the true nature of universal illnesses: first, the way we *label* conditions in different settings, and second, how conditions are *expressed* in different cultures.

Labelling

As Leff's butterfly example shows, two people in different settings may look at the same thing and give it two different names. Within the psychiatric field, it was at one time thought that there was a higher rate of schizophrenia in the USA than in Britain. When the method of diagnosis was standardized in the two countries, however, apparently large differences disappeared (Cooper et al., 1972). Psychiatrists in the USA, seeing the same patient as psychiatrists from Britain, were more likely to diagnose schizophrenia than were the British psychiatrists, who were more likely to diagnose a mood disorder. This early research gave rise to an important approach to thinking about and refining psychiatric diagnosis, which will be discussed in more detail in Chapter 3.

Expression of distress

As we shall see later in this book, the emphasis in Western culture on describing distress psychologically is not shared by every culture. In many parts of the world, including Africa, there is a tendency for personal distress to be expressed as bodily pains and problems. A universalist would try to determine whether those experiencing these pains and problems are suffering from what a Western psychiatrist would call depression. Universalists attempt to strip off the layers of cultural casing. They wish to show, for example, that a person complaining of shoulder pain in Harare, say, with no organic reason for the pain, or who complains of thinking too much (Abas et al., 1994), and who does not complain about psychological problems, may be just as depressed as someone in London who complains of depression. Both may get better on a course of antidepressants.

This approach to understanding mental illness cross-culturally has the value of making the world knowable to us. If only we can crack the codes of different ways of talking about mental illness, and different ways of expressing it, we can study mental illness the world over. The universalist tradition has given rise to major studies such as the International Pilot Study of Schizophrenia (WHO, 1973, 1979), which explored schizophrenia in a number of countries across the world. A single diagnostic system, and the assumption that the disorder being studied was the same, enabled the researchers to ask and answer questions about how common schizophrenia is in different cultures, and whether the outcome differs across cultures. The methodology of such studies is essentially quantitative – it involves the counting of symptoms and events. It also allows for easy comparison across a range of contexts.

Universalism as practised in Western psychiatry tends to use Western diagnostic systems as the standard. Implicit in this approach is the belief that Western psychiatry has discovered the core syndromes, and different manifestations in different parts of the world are unusual versions of these syndromes. Clearly, this view does not give equal weight and value to all ways of seeing the world. A further feature of the approach is that it tends to look at disorders as existing 'out there' to be discovered – like Leff's butterflies. It does not give careful attention to the notion that our ways of seeing the world, and our assumptions, help shape how we see the world. Mental illnesses, to varying degrees, are viewed as things and not as processes which happen both to people and between people. Viewing mental illness as a thing is an example of what is known as *reification* – a process of viewing social relationships as fixed and static entities.

2 Relativism

In 1977, Kleinman defined a major direction in the field of culture and mental health when he attacked universalist psychiatry, calling it the 'old transcultural psychiatry', and proposed a relativist alternative, which he termed the 'new cross-cultural psychiatry'. Some of his criticisms have been anticipated in the above argument. His most damning critique, though, was probably in his calling the 'old transcultural psychiatry' a form of 'veterinary psychiatry'. By this, Kleinman meant that universalist psychiatry, far from actually being universal, simply imposed Western psychiatric models on the world, and did not take sufficient account of the actual experience of suffering. By looking only for a limited range of signs and symptoms which could be elicited quite easily, universalists were not entering into the emotional worlds of the people they were studying and treating, and were practising a science similar to that of a veterinarian – a person who works with animals.

In support of a relativist approach informed by anthropology, Kleinman raised the important distinction which has been made in medical anthropology and medical sociology between *disease* and *illness*. At that time, Kleinman wrote of disease as the malfunctioning of the body, and illness as the lived experience of suffering. According to him, it is not enough to understand the physical disease of any person, though this may be universal. What is equally important is the person's experience of illness and distress, as it is this experience which will determine how the person behaves, the treatment sought, and the reaction to treatment. There have been many different definitions of disease and illness, but what they have in common is the view that there are different ways of understanding mental suffering. In short, disease can be seen to stand for the doctor's perspective on disorder, and illness for the patient's perspective. These may be very different. For example, a doctor may believe a patient has a brain tumour (disease), but the patient may believe that bewitchment is at work (illness). Unless the doctor takes account of this different view, there may be serious consequences for treatment. For example, life-saving surgery may be refused by someone who does not see the need for it in terms of the illness perspective.

How does one deal, as a practitioner, with these differences in perspective? The first and most important thing is to be aware of them. Many beliefs which patients hold may seem strange or odd to mental health workers, but these beliefs have their own internal logic, and can affect the patient's future dramatically. Simply recognizing and respecting this diversity is likely to improve the relationship between the practitioner and the client. Kleinman and his colleagues (Katon & Kleinman, 1981; Kleinman, 1988; Kleinman et al., 1978) have developed a systematic way of asking about patients' illness experiences, an approach which is now associated with a large research tradition (Weiss, 1997). They speak of *explanatory models*, which are the ways in which we all understand our own illnesses. When people become ill, they argue, they always ask the following questions (though not necessarily consciously):

- Why me?
- Why now?
- What is wrong?
- How long will it last and how serious is it?
- What problems does it create for me?
- How do I get rid of this problem? That is, what will make me better? (Kleinman, 1988: 156)

The job of the clinician is not only to understand the patient's explanatory model, but also to negotiate between the professional explanatory model and that held by the patient, so that there can be some common ground and a basis for treatment which will be acceptable to both. If, for example, a primary health care nurse is treating a patient for what he or she believes to be depression, but what the patient may believe is a serious, life-threatening, physical illness, the treatment will not be acceptable to the patient until there has been some discussion of why the nurse is acting as he or she is. A common understanding is likely to increase the extent to which the patient participates in treatment by following advice, taking medication, and so on. One of the major problems facing every form of health care is the question of whether patients follow the treatments suggested – this is known as *compliance* or *adherence* – and negotiating between explanatory models, it is argued, increases the possibility of compliance or adherence.

A special challenge is faced by practitioners when there is illness in the absence of disease or disease in the absence of illness. Anybody who has worked in a primary health care setting will have come across the frustrating patient who believes himself or herself to be ill but who has no pathology on examination. Having a relativist perspective helps us get away from our simple frustration and irritation and realize that, for whatever reason – this may be cultural, social, psychological, or a combination – the person *is* experiencing an illness. There may be no disease, and we may have no way of helping the person within our health system, but we do not question the person's own reality or simply give a label of troublemaker. This attitude of respect and curiosity about what may be troubling the person may be very helpful in itself in finding other avenues for the person to get help.

The alternative – where there is disease but no illness – can be equally challenging. Consider the case of a man with a brain tumour. This man collapsed one day at work, without there having been any warning signs. He woke up in a hospital bed, not remembering anything that had happened, and experiencing no pain or other symptoms. To add to the problem, nobody on the staff could speak his language, and he couldn't speak theirs. Nobody explained to him why he was there, and he felt quite well. It was hardly surprising that he decided he wanted to leave the hospital immediately. In that situation, a discussion in his own language which explained in some detail what had happened, and what the professionals' explanatory model was, was essential.

Until now, I have been writing as though patient explanatory models and practitioner explanatory models always come from different cultural universes, and are completely different. This is, of course, rarely the case, as will be seen in later chapters. Adding further confusion is the possibility that patients and practitioners may be using the same words to discuss different things. There are particular challenges when we deal with chronic illnesses and psychiatric illnesses in particular. For example, most of us who have been exposed to biomedicine are used to medicine being used mainly to treat symptoms – to make someone feel better. But some medicines are used for prophylaxis – that is, for the prevention of symptoms, or of relapse of a condition. Prophylactic medications are often to be taken when the person feels quite well. People with major mood disturbance problems may be put on a long-term course of lithium carbonate, which helps prevent further mood problems. A significant proportion of these will stop taking the lithium when their mood feels stable, as it feels strange to take medicine when you are feeling well. There are, of course, other reasons why patients may stop taking medicine – apart from anything else, it is very unpleasant to be reminded daily that you have a chronic illness when you are feeling fine – but one of them may be that the concept of taking medication for prophylaxis is foreign.

A major public health problem is that of hypertension (high blood pressure). Hypertension is another condition for which medication may have to be taken even when the person feels quite well. This medication may be essential to prevent serious consequences such as strokes. In the case of hypertension, there is the added challenge that the name for the condition uses a word which many of us associate with psychological states of tension. Blumhagen (1982) showed that some people with hypertension interpreted the condition as hypertension – or increased emotional tension. Such people may be more likely to take their hypertension medication when they feel emotionally upset and not to take it when feeling calm. This would have important implications for the management of the disease, and if this problem is anticipated by the clinician, it has more chance of being avoided.

A further example of the importance of understanding different models and ways of using language can be seen from a South African study of epilepsy in an Afrikaans-speaking community. After the study was completed (McQueen & Swartz, 1995), the chief researcher and her colleagues held a workshop for community members to discuss the results. They had expected that there would be a stigma associated with epilepsy (as has been found with other studies all over the world), but what they had not realized was that part of the stigma in this context came from the (French) name for different types of seizures – grand mal and petit mal. The word *mal* in Afrikaans means 'mad', and people in this community thought that if they suffered from petit mal or grand mal seizures, this meant that they were being labelled as a little mad or very mad. This is exactly the opposite of what people working in the field of epilepsy are trying to promote – they are trying to educate the public that epilepsy is *not* a form of mental illness. This example would be amusing if the labels and their interpretation in this community had not had such serious implications for epileptics and their families.

In trying to understand illness experiences in different contexts, relativists gain as full a picture as possible of the meaning of the illness to the sufferer, in the context of the sufferer's own family, community, and spiritual background. An approach to knowledge which is interested in meaning is known as a *hermeneutic* approach, and there is a focus on obtaining *qualitative* data as opposed to counts of numbers of symptoms, and so on. Relativists try to find out as much as possible about how people's lives shape their illnesses and how their illnesses affect their lives.

Potential difficulties with relativism

Many relativist studies provide rich information on practices and beliefs in local contexts. The scope of these studies tends to be small, and there is more emphasis on understanding what is happening locally than on making broad cross-national comparisons. A study such as the International Pilot Study of Schizophrenia would not have been possible in this model, and quick, easy cross-national comparisons are not possible. In extreme cases, relativists would argue that no comparisons across contexts are possible, as meanings differ in these different places. This view could lead to knowledge which is quite fragmented and difficult to organize.

This is indeed a potential disadvantage of a relativist approach. The desire to be as true to context as possible may cause relativists to lose the big picture. But, relativists would argue, it is important to see that the Western diagnostic systems are themselves cultural products, and though it may be easy to view the world in terms of these systems, this is not necessarily the best or most useful way of seeing the world. Kim and Berry (1993) argue that relativism may offer the chance to look at universals in a different way. In putting forward this view, they draw on what is known as the emic/etic distinction. The term *etic* has been used to describe a universalist approach which imposes a particular way of seeing the world (generally, Western) on the data observed. An *emic* approach, by contrast, looks at the world-view of the people being studied and sees this as central. Kim and Berry (1993) believe it is possible to conduct a series of emic studies in different cultures and then to explore what commonalities exist between these cultures. In this way, it is possible to reach a universal understanding across these cultures – what these authors call a *derived etic* – which is different from what they call the *imposed etic*, which usually comes from the imposition of Western norms on non-Western cultures. The key difference is that in the case of a derived etic, any universals will emerge from a series of local studies and not from assumptions held by researchers before they conduct the studies. We may, of course, debate the extent to which the ideal of a derived etic is possible. We can also question the extent to which researchers' or clinicians' assumptions about the world can be removed from any consideration of how the world works, as we have seen from the work of Clifford (1986) cited earlier in this chapter.

A second potential difficulty with relativist studies in the field of mental health is that they may not be easy to use clinically. For example, many relativist studies explore modes of healing in non-Western settings. The information provided may be interesting, but will not necessarily give the Western, biomedically-trained practitioner pointers as to how to work. This is not in itself a criticism of relativist approaches – many who write in this area are not concerned with how to change Western clinical practice. But it can lead some clinicians to lack patience with relativist studies. Often, there is much that can be learned clinically from reading about how healing happens in other cultures, and it is also certainly true that the hermeneutic approach favoured by relativists has much to offer Western practice (cf. Murphy, 1977). It may be short-sighted to expect all research to be immediately of use and applicable in the biomedical context, as good research should help one think, and thinking about what people may need and experience will impact on clinical work. The impatience that some may have, though, with relativism and its lack of quick answers and guidelines for action must lead us to the question of why we study mental health and illness cross-culturally. This is the starting point for critical approaches to the field.

3 Critical approaches

Why do we study cultural factors in mental health and illness? There are many answers to this question, and none is the single 'right' answer. I myself am a South African clinical psychologist. I am interested in the provision of appropriate mental health services to all people, and I am also interested in the roles that communities and people of all kinds contribute to mental health and, regrettably, to suffering as well. If I were an anthropologist with a special interest in ritual, though, I might be studying the field in order to come to a clearer understanding of the social function of ritual in different parts of the world. If I were a pharmacologist, I might want to know how drugs and drug-taking behaviour differ in different contexts, and what these variations might imply for the international pharmaceutical industry. If I were a faith healer, I might be interested in finding out what academic research says in support of alternative healing systems. The possibilities are almost endless.

Critical approaches to the culture and mental health field are not separate from other approaches, nor are they unified in how they deal with the area. But a key factor common to critical approaches is that they all ask why knowledge is produced, and in whose interests. For example, as we shall see in Chapter 8, Young (1980, 1995) has shown how much of our understanding of 'stress' relates to issues faced by the USA after the Vietnam War. Scheper-Hughes (1992) argues that infant death in Brazil, and the way that it is thought about internationally, has links with international and local socioeconomic issues. Sharp (1980) and Thornton (1988) demonstrate the links between academic writing on culture in South Africa in the 1980s and previously, and apartheid ideology.

Taking a critical position with respect to transcultural psychiatry in Britain, Littlewood and Lipsedge (1997) have argued that the proper business of research in this field is not simply to explore cultural factors in mental health, but also to engage actively in building what they term an anti-racist psychiatry. Elsewhere, Littlewood (1988) argues that close analysis even of the way a particular diagnosis is made in British psychiatry – that of toxic psychosis – demonstrates racist practice (see Chapter 10). Furthermore, Littlewood and Lipsedge (1997) recall that in the USA at the time of slavery, there was a psychiatric condition known as drapetomania. This condition described the irresistible urge some slaves had to run away! If psychiatric diagnosis can have been used in such a flagrantly oppressive manner in the past, it is possible that the same thing can be happening now. Psychotherapy as a practice may appear to be more benign and less dangerous than other aspects of mental health practice, but this is not necessarily true. Introducing a text on intercultural therapy, Littlewood (1992b:13) describes psychotherapy as potentially an 'insidious ... agent of social control', and calls on readers to be aware of this at all times.

There is an extensive literature on the effects of racism and oppression on mental health and also on mental health practices and practitioners acting in an oppressive manner both in terms of the way patients are treated at times and in the way that psychiatric knowledge is produced. An important part of this literature is work which explores the psychology of oppression from the point of view of the oppressed – whether the oppression be racist, sexist, based on religion, social class, or any other social category. Fanon (1970), a psychiatrist working in Algeria, wrote a classic account of the effects of oppression on identity formation and development in Africa. This theme was taken up in South Africa by Biko (1978) and explored more fully from a psychological perspective by Manganyi (1973). More recently, black South African psychologists have explored questions of the psychological consequences of oppression in more detail (Nicholas, 1993; Nicholas & Cooper, 1990), and the potential for mental health practitioners to contribute to national healing and reconstruction is being explored.

Many of these issues will be returned to in more detail in Chapter 8. Entire books have been devoted to critical questions about mental health but we cannot consider all of these in detail. At this stage, however, it is important that we keep asking questions about what is being said, and why, in the knowledge we create about culture and mental health. Who is writing about whom, and why? Are some of the debates that we shall be looking at more about those who are writing them than about the people who use mental health services? These and other questions are central if we are to understand cultural issues in the mental health field. It is clear that cultural factors and issues of power affect people's lives and the ways that these lives are discussed and brought to the attention of people like you – the readers of this book.

Conclusion

This chapter has dealt with some of the ways we approach questions surrounding the interrelationship between culture and mental health. We began by looking at some definitions and then considered different traditions of approaching the field. All approaches have their strengths and weaknesses, and it will be your task as a reader to develop your own understanding and approach as you go through this book. What should be clear by now is that there is no one correct way of looking at things, and that evidence which is presented in this book (or any book) is not simply 'the truth'. Your job as a reader is to read actively and critically – to make up your own mind. You may not always agree with me. This is a good thing. I hope that in the chapters that follow you will think actively, disagree where you do disagree, and develop your own approach to this complex and fascinating field.

PART II

Finding out about mental
health and illness

2

Language diversity and mental health care

SOME YEARS AGO, I was conducting research in a large general hospital in Cape Town. One day, when I was observing practices in the
psychiatric emergency unit (see Swartz, 1992), a strange scene developed, which encapsulated for me some key issues we need to think
about when considering the role of language in mental health care.

I was sitting in on interviews of patients conducted by a psychiatric
registrar (a psychiatrist in training). The registrar called a patient into
his office, but soon realized that the patient could not speak English,
and he, the registrar, could not speak Xhosa, the patient's language.
The registrar called in a relative of the patient to interpret. It soon
became clear, though, that the relative did not speak very good
English himself, and he was having difficulty translating back and
forth from English into Xhosa and vice versa. Clearly, the registrar
needed another interpreter, so he called in the Xhosa-speaking ward
cleaner. He did not, however, wish to be rude to the relative so he
allowed him to stay for the remainder of the interview. The interview
now proceeded as follows: the registrar would ask a question of the
cleaner in English, the cleaner would ask the same question of the
relative (but in Xhosa), the relative would repeat the Xhosa question
to the patient, the patient would reply in Xhosa to the relative, the
relative would repeat the Xhosa reply to the cleaner, the cleaner
would give the reply in English to the registrar, and the registrar
would the write the translated reply into the patient's file. Then the
registrar would ask the next question, and the process would start

again. As all this was going on, I was in the corner taking notes and, as it happened, the hospital was being rebuilt, so there were loud crashing noises throughout, and much of the interview had to be conducted with all participants shouting above the din.

After some time, the registrar came to the part of the assessment interview where orientation is assessed. This assessment is designed to give an insight into cognitive functioning of the patient, and helps the clinician to decide whether the patient is suffering from an organic brain syndrome. The questioning, through the interpreting of the cleaner and the relative, at first followed the standard questions. 'Who are you?' asked the registrar, and the patient responded correctly through the interpreters. 'Where are you?' – a similar correct response. 'What day is it today?' – again, a correct response. The registrar had established that the patient was oriented for person, place, and time. Then, the registrar asked a non-standard question: 'Who am I?' This question was relayed to the patient through the cleaner and the relative, and the answer came back through the relative and the cleaner: 'You are a secretary'. The registrar turned to me, and said, rather drily, 'At last – a patient who understands what my real job is!'

This scene demonstrates many of the difficulties mental health services face in a multilingual context. The image of the psychiatric interview as an intimate relationship between the distressed patient on the one hand, and the caring, empathic psychiatrist on the other, is shattered. The issue of confidentiality, a value held dear in biomedicine, and mental health services in particular, is raised when relatives and ward cleaners are used as interpreters (at times, other patients serve as interpreters as well). The patient in the scene above was quite correct in viewing the psychiatric interview conducted under the above circumstances as essentially administrative rather than healing encounters.

A scene like the above one is familiar to just about everybody working in the mental health field in multilingual contexts, in South Africa certainly. At the same time, though, if one examines the international and the South African literature on culture and mental health, the language issue is not given much prominence.

For example, the recently published *World mental health* (Desjarlais et al., 1995) makes almost no mention of language issues in the design and provision of services in low-income countries. Recently, I sought advice from colleagues in an electronic discussion group for a chapter on language and mental health. Some responded by saying that I should not be focusing on language at all, but on culture in general. In examining cross-cultural psychiatry under apartheid many years ago, a colleague and I commented that it is perhaps easier to focus broadly on cultural issues than on the specifics of how interviewers need to be able to communicate with patients and their families (Swartz & Foster, 1984). Language is the basis of most assessments in mental health care, and is central to almost all forms of treatment. Even drug treatments need to be discussed with and understood by patients, if patients are to take the drugs prescribed. In this chapter we shall be looking at the challenges that language diversity poses not only for mental health practice, but for research as well. We shall begin by looking very briefly at theories of language, and then at the clinical interview using an interpreter, and what this interview can tell us both about language and broader cultural issues in mental health care.

Theories of language

The question of how language relates to our thoughts and emotions is very complex. Does language simply reflect our thoughts and feelings? Does language construct our thoughts and feelings? Is it possible to have thoughts and feelings without language? Questions such as these have occupied, and continue to occupy, the research of philosophers, linguists, psychologists, and many others. For the purposes of this chapter, however, we shall simply contrast two basic approaches to understanding how language works. Good and Good (1980) contrast the *empiricist* theory of language with the *hermeneutic* approach to language.

The empiricist approach to language

In this view, language refers to things, and serves only as a way of labelling the reality 'out there'. This implies that different languages are no more than different sets of labels for realities which are common across the world. This view is reflected in the example of Leff's butterfly collectors in Chapter 1. The difficulty the collectors had with communication about the butterflies was essentially that of finding common labels for the same things.

The empiricist approach to language is very pragmatic. Translation, in this model, is the search for appropriate labels for entities which exist in the world. The best translation is one that provides labels in two languages which refer to exactly the same things – like the same butterflies.

This view of language was satirized by Jonathan Swift in his novel *Gulliver's travels*, first published in 1726 (Swift, 1965). Swift describes a society in which words are seen to be things, and his characters decide it would be easier to communicate without language, by simply showing things to one another. The members of Swift's society walk around with large sacks on their backs, showing off different things to one another. This absurd picture of people trying to be mute while showing one another things from their bags was used by Swift to support his view that language was both more complex and more powerful than simply a set of labels for things.

The hermeneutic / constructionist approach to language

According to this approach, language plays a part in the construction of meaning. Language 'creates' its own reality; we negotiate reality through language. Our feelings are affected and shaped by the words we use and the vocabulary and sentence construction we have available to us. Translation in this model is a complicated matter – it involves not simply changing labels for things in the world, but also a consideration of the role language plays in determining our emotional realities. In her moving account of the experience of adolescence in a culture and language very different from those she was born into, Hoffman (1989) describes herself as *Lost in translation* (the title of her autobiography). People who are brought up bilingual, furthermore, commonly speak of some emotions being better expressed in some languages than in others. We also know that different languages develop different systems of vocabulary for emotions, and in different ways. For example, in Xhosa, the word *ububele* can be used to mean either 'emotion' or 'kindness' – quite separate words in English. Interestingly, the word *ububele* is derived from the Xhosa word for the female breast – *ibele* – which gives us some idea of the connotations of this feeling word in Xhosa.

There are many other examples of ways in which translation of emotional terminology involves more than a simple change of labels for a single thing, and these will appear again and again throughout this book. There remain, though, questions about how to interpret differences across languages in words used for distress. When we are told, for example, that the words 'depression' and 'anxiety' have no direct equivalents in the Nigerian language Yoruba (Leff, 1988: 43), do we conclude that depression and anxiety do not exist amongst the Yoruba people? If the Chinese have only one word for 'anxiety', 'tension', and 'worrying', then what does this tell us about emotional experience in China? These questions suggest large research enterprises in themselves. In considering the issue of depression cross-culturally, Lutz (1985) talks of 'depression and the translation of emotional worlds', and suggests that the apparently simple act of trying to determine how many depressed people there are in various cultures raises questions about how we all see and categorize the world.

In summary, then, if we hold the *empiricist* view, the task of translating is simply finding the appropriate words in different languages for feeling states. If on the other hand we hold the *hermeneutic/constructionist* view, the task of translating is more complex: we have to consider the extent to which the act of translation implies the construction of a particular reality.

The interpreted interview

Let us now consider what happens in an interview where an interpreter is present. As we shall see, this interview can be analysed at a variety of levels, the first of which is the interpersonal level.

The interpersonal level

When there is an interpreter present, it is obvious that an interview between two people has now become a situation in which there are three people present. Not only this – two of the people in this triangle cannot communicate with each other (the interviewer and the patient). This means that all communication between them will be routed through the interpreter. From research on couple therapy, we know that where there is a triangle, alliances are likely to form between two parties in the triangle, implicitly against the third person (Haley, 1976). Given that the interviewer and the patient cannot communicate direct-ly with each other, the chances are that alliances that may develop will be either between the interpreter and the patient, or between the inter-preter and the interviewer. These alliances may, of course, shift and change through the interview, and may not be nearly as hostile as the term 'alliance' may imply. But the possibility of them immediately raises the question of whose agent the interpreter is. Is the interpreter there for the interviewer or for the patient?

At first glance, this may seem to be an absurd question. The inter-preter, surely, is there for *both* the interviewer *and* the patient – to make sure they understand each other. The reality is, though, that an inter-preter is not and can never be simply a kind of dictionary or telephone exchange through which people can communicate. An interpreter, like the interviewer and the patient, is a person with feelings, beliefs, and desires. The interpreter may feel close to the patient by virtue of being able to speak the patient's language and possibly coming from the same social background as the patient. Conversely, the interpreter may feel close to the interviewer by being part of the mental health team. Different interpreters at different times may feel like the agent of the interviewer or the agent of the patient or, indeed, interpreters may have a range of different agendas and beliefs about their roles. This leads us to the next level of understanding how interpreting works.

The institutional level

The reasons for using an interpreter are not simply interpersonal – they also relate to the institution and its needs. The hospital I discussed at the beginning of this chapter, for example, had no staff high in the mental health hierarchy (psychologists or psychiatrists) who could speak Xhosa. There were also no posts for interpreters at the hospital then. This raises questions about the hospital's commitment, at that time, to equal care for all its patients. In fact, there are a number of mental health facilities which exclude clients from certain services on the basis of language alone – for example, group therapies are run only in certain languages. If an institution providing mental health services does not have a policy working to address the needs of all its clients, to ensure equal access to care for all clients, this impacts on the interpreting relationship.

For example, when the institution has no other plan in place and so interviewers are forced at times to use relatives as interpreters, these relatives may want to present to the interviewers as good an impression as possible of their relatives. Alternatively, some relatives may be so concerned to convince the clinician of how bad things are at home, that they may want the clinician to have an extremely bad impression of the relative. Where a cleaner is used, he or she may regard the chance to interpret as an honour, for example, or an extra unpaid workload, a privilege or an infringement on her or his rights in terms of industrial relations. All these different institutional interpretations will affect how the interpreter works. Similarly, the clinician may feel angry with the institution for allowing a situation in which ad hoc arrangements have to be made for interpreting, or the clinician may feel inadequate working this way, or irritated at the cleaner's lack of skill in interpreting. All of these factors will impact on the interview in different ways. The client will probably also have feelings about the use of interpreters, and this will also affect how the interview progresses.

In South African hospitals it is reasonably common for nursing staff to be used as interpreters for medical personnel – as it is in many other parts of the world. Since multilingual nursing staff – particularly professional nurses – are generally employed for their nursing skills, not the languages they speak, what happens to the institutional role of the nurse who is called upon to interpret?

First, there is a problem with the way the nurse's *expertise* is seen – is the nurse in this role viewed primarily as a clinician in his or her own right, or is the nurse now being used simply as a way for the doctor or psychologist to gain access to the patient? There may be a denial of aspects of the competence of the nurse as a clinician in her or his own right, with clinical skills to contribute. I saw an aspect of this being played out when I was observing case discussions ('ward rounds') in a large psychiatric hospital some years ago (Swartz, 1991a). A highly competent professional nurse was called upon to interpret for a psychiatrist. This the professional nurse did, and very competently. At the same time, though, when the professional nurse did not agree with the way in which the psychiatrist was conducting the interview, she simply asked her own questions of the patient, and then gave the clinician the answers she thought the psychiatrist needed to hear. The psychiatrist, of course, was unaware of this as she could not understand what was passing between the patient and the nurse. As it happens, the patients were well served by what may be termed resistance on the professional nurse's part to the constraints of the interpreting role (cf. Drennan et al., 1991) as the professional nurse was very skilled clinically. Nevertheless, recognition of expertise (or lack of it) remains a problem.

The interpreter's role, in keeping with a hermeneutic view of language, is often seen as more than that of someone to provide the correct words. The interpreter is viewed as a *culture broker*, who can inform the interviewer about the cultural background and assumptions of the client. This seems very sensible, but can create problems in the institutional context, in which it is often assumed that the nurse, because she can speak the patient's language, also understands and is able to portray sympathetically the cultural background of the client. The nurse may not identify with the client's beliefs at all and, in fact, may be opposed to many of them, especially those beliefs concerning different healing systems. The nurse is put in the position of having a *transitional status* between the world of biomedicine and that of the patient. This is well and good if the nurse feels that this status is a correct ascription, but many nurses may not. In this context, there may be a denial of aspects of the *identity* of the nurse as interpreter, within the institution. Nurses, for example, may consider themselves fully part of the world of the doctor, and not people who, in a sense, have to stand in for the world of the patient. This problem with role and identity may be felt by any person who in their work is assumed to 'stand for' a whole group of people – for example, the only woman on a work team, the only Jew, and so on. What is especially ironical in this situation is that in multilingual countries, where clinicians cannot communicate with their clients directly, the clients often represent the majority in those countries. This leads us to explore the next level of analysis of the interpreted interview.

The socio-political level

Some readers may be feeling justifiably irritated with my focus on interpreters. Surely the problem in mental health care can best be solved by employing people who can communicate directly with their patients. This is, of course, true, but the reality is that in many parts of the world personnel in the higher echelons of mental health care do not speak all the indigenous languages. This state of affairs has arisen as a result of a number of factors, including limited access to higher education for members of all language groups. This is compounded by the fact that proficiency in indigenous languages is often not valued or necessary as part of the competency of a clinician.

South Africa is an especially interesting case in this regard. Currently, there are eleven official languages in South Africa, but prior to the inception of democracy in 1994 there were only two – English and Afrikaans. South Africa's long history of struggle between the British and the Boers (dating back well over 150 years) ensured that for a long time the issue of language was central in political conflicts. As long ago as the 1940s, around the time that the National Party, representing Afrikaner interests, came to power and instituted apartheid, language issues between English and Afrikaans were strongly felt within the nursing profession (Marks, 1994). Educational policies under National Party rule ensured that clinicians (as well as others) could in general converse in Afrikaans, making services accessible to Afrikaans-speakers. In addition, education policies ensured that high quality education and tertiary education were more readily available to whites than to others – and whites generally have Afrikaans and/or English as home languages. Other language groups, being black, were largely sidelined. We can see therefore that whereas the practice of a profession like psychiatry was dominated by English-speakers in the nineteenth century, by the latter half of this century not only were the majority of services accessible to Afrikaans-speakers, but Afrikaans-speakers were in major positions of power in the mental health field. This shows how an aggressive language policy can radically change the accessibility of services based on language – and it also shows how policies can help keep services relatively inaccessible to members of other language groups.

There is no doubt, therefore, that part of what happens in an interpreted interview has to do with political factors. In low-income countries with a colonial history, the chances are that the power relationship of colonizer versus colonized is to a degree mirrored by the relationship between clinician and client, with the interpreter being somewhere in between, presenting the colonized world of the client for the benefit of the work of the clinician. This power relationship impacts on the interview. It is a very different role, for example, for a Shona-speaking nurse in Zimbabwe to be interpreting for a white Zimbabwean psychiatrist than it is for a French-speaking nurse to be interpreting for an English-speaking psychiatrist in Britain who has a French patient on a ward. The history of colonialism and the current postcolonial situation is different in the two cases.

If there are to be changes to the situation where clinical interviews have to be mediated through interpreters, there will invariably have to be broader political changes. Later in the chapter we will discuss some suggestions that have been made in thinking about broad language policies which can affect access to mental health services. In the next section, though, we will look briefly at the international context for concern about language and mental health care.

The international level

As I have mentioned earlier, the spread of psychiatry and other mental health specialities internationally has been associated with the spread of colonialism. Psychiatry is a Western product, as we saw in the previous chapter. For this reason, psychiatric practices in Africa and many other parts of the world have been associated with the concerns and interests of colonizers. Over the years, this has affected language policies in the professions, and the ability of professionals to converse in a variety of indigenous languages. This pattern is reflected in similar patterns in biomedicine and more generally in colonial contexts.

Global changes in the twentieth century have also affected language issues in mental health care. There are an unprecedented number of refugees in the world at present, and huge migrations as a consequence of war, famine, oppression, and other problems. These global shifts have led to an influx of clients in the mental health systems of many developed countries. The issues of interpreting are therefore as relevant to a monolingual psychologist working in South Africa, for example, as they are to a monolingual psychologist in Australia working with South-East Asian refugees. Obviously, there are differences in the local politics surrounding what happens in the interviews, but both interpreting experiences are affected by global and international issues.

In the context of a world of great mobility and where there are so many refugees, there is probably no practitioner anywhere in the world who will not at some time have to confront the issue of language differences in mental health work. The ideal, always, of course, is to have clinicians available who can converse directly with clients. Given that this is not always possible, it is important that everyone interested in cultural factors in mental health care – indeed, that everyone interested in mental health care – have some understanding of what is at stake in an interpreting relationship. This applies as much to those who are likely to use the services of interpreters as to those who are likely to be interpreters. In the next section, therefore, we shall look at some of the technical issues involving interviews where interpreters are employed.

Technical aspects of interpreting

How should an interpreter and someone who uses an interpreter best behave in a clinical interview? Simply asking the question in this way implies a certain approach to the issue. All too often, clinicians do not realize that both the interpreter and the person using the interpreter need to understand the clinical interpreting triangle, and to develop their work accordingly. Clinicians may complain that they are already skilled in mental health interviewing and that they do not need to learn how to work with interpreters – any adjustments that need to be made must be made by the interpreter and not by the interviewer. Though this is clearly not true, it is a view which gives us insight into one of the common views of the interpreter role.

Different views of the interpreter role

The invisible interpreter

The most obvious view of interpreters is that they should act simply as channels to clients, and should be invisible in the process. Whatever the interviewer says should be conveyed directly to the patient by the interpreter, and the client's words should be conveyed back to the interviewer – hence the *invisible interpreter*. This model is often unconsciously assumed to be the correct one, especially by clinicians who have not thought about interpreting very carefully. It is also consistent with the empiricist view of language – the interpreter's job is simply to remove the labels of one language and affix the labels of another.

Interpreter as culture broker

As mentioned earlier, interpreters are often called upon to be *culture brokers* for the interviewers they work with. In order to assess mental illness and distress, one needs to know whether a patient's beliefs are in keeping with the group he or she comes from. For example, in some societies, to explain misfortune in terms of bewitchment is the cultural norm; in others this explanation may be so unusual as to suggest the possibility of mental illness. Where the interpreter is seen as a culture broker, he or she will be called upon to help the clinician make an assessment in situations such as these. The interpreter will also explain to the interviewer the context and meaning of aspects of the patient's life – for

example, the interpreter may explain to the clinician what the significance of an initiation ritual might have been for a patient. The culture
broker role may also be important in helping the clinician make assessments of the patient's behaviour during the interview. An interpreter
may be asked, for example, whether the patient's not making eye
contact with the clinician is a culturally appropriate sign of respect (as it
is in certain cultures) or a way of avoiding the clinician (Gillis et al., 1982;
Swartz et al., 1985).

We have already considered some of the difficulties that interpreters may face in being seen as culture brokers, and it is not realistic
to expect any interpreter to understand fully the cultural background
of every person the clinician deals with. But a person able to speak the
client's language may often know more about the client's cultural
background than the clinician who cannot converse with the client.

Interpreter as junior colleague

When an interpreter is acting as a culture broker, he or she is already
making judgements about the patient – and these judgements are
often clinical judgements (for example, Is this belief culturally acceptable or a sign of mental illness?). If interpreters have had training in the
health or mental health field, they will inevitably bring their own skills
to bear on the interview. In the case of any mental health assessment,
furthermore, clinicians are often interested not only in the content of
what is being said but also in the way it is being said – what psychiatrists
call the form of talk. Some psychotic people talk in such a way that it is
almost impossible to repeat what they say word for word, let alone to
translate what they have said into another language. In such a situation, it takes some skill for an interpreter to recognize and to be able to
convey to the clinician whether there is simply a problem with the
content of the talk or with the way the person is talking. Judgements
are necessary in less extreme situations as well – for example, in assessing whether a person is talking unusually slowly and deliberately or
unusually quickly. These are easy to see where the difference in speech
pattern is very far from the norm, but are more difficult to assess when
the pattern is subtly different from what is usual.

Viewing the interpreter as a junior colleague involves recognizing the skills the good interpreter brings to the interview and using these skills in a team approach, where the interpreter's opinions form part of the team judgement about the client. This involves working with the interpreter in a very different way from, for example, working with an interpreter whom the clinician would like to regard as invisible. The case may be discussed with the interpreter both before and after the interview. At specific points during the interview the clinician and the interpreter may wish to discuss what the patient is saying and how to approach the rest of the interview. This may assist both in gaining the most accurate and clinically useful picture of the client, but due regard needs to be taken of how it may feel for the client to be discussed in the third person while being present in the room, and practices must be adjusted in accordance with what is humane and comfortable for the client.

The *junior colleague* model of the interpreter goes further than either of the previous models in recognizing the skills and importance of the interpreter. But if the interpreter's skills are so central to the interview, why is the interpreter seen as a *junior* colleague? This is a legitimate question, which I shall return to later in the chapter.

Interpreter as client advocate

In this model, the interpreter is employed specifically to look after the interests of the client. Clients, it is argued, and especially clients who cannot speak the dominant language of the institution, are in a far less powerful position than are the clinicians. The interpreter role, then, is to assist the client with access to resources – essentially to empower the client. This may involve the interpreter in a more ongoing and intimate relationship with the client and those close to him or her. In fact, by the time the clinician comes to interview the client, the interpreter may already know the client quite well and have some ideas as to how she or he can best access the institution's resources. This model of interpreting is also sometimes known as the *community interpreting* approach, because of its emphasis on community needs and questions of power relationships across communities.

Common errors

Vasquez and Javier (1991: 163) describe a psychiatric interview where a patient who has taken an overdose of medication says 'Just tell the doctor I took the pills by mistake'. Her 15-year-old nephew, who is interpreting for her, tells the doctor that his aunt 'was only trying to sleep and she thought that the medication would help'. Similarly, Muller (1994) describes serious errors in an interview when an interpreter is used in a busy South African psychiatric hospital. For example, a patient describes his interactions with peers in quite some detail and, possibly to spare the patient the pain of having this information explored by the psychiatrist, the interpreter relays that the patient does not wish to speak about relationships with peers.

According to Vasquez and Javier (1991), the most common mistakes made by interpreters include:

1 *Omission* – occurs when the interpreter leaves out part or all of a message sent by one of the people speaking. This can happen especially when there is a large amount of content in the interview and the interpreter starts leaving out parts of what has been said.

2 *Addition* – occurs when the interpreter adds to what the speaker has said, often to clarify matters or to make the interview flow more smoothly or politely. This can be a problem especially when the interviewer has specific questions or instructions for the client but these are added to by the interpreter and the interviewer does not know this is happening. It can invalidate any assessment of intellectual functioning, for example.

3 *Condensation* – is a very common problem, where the interpreter summarizes what has been said according to the interpreter's own views as to what is important in the interview. These views may differ significantly from those of both the interviewer and the client. Every clinician who has worked with an interpreter when neither has been properly prepared will have had the experience of the interpreter and the client having a long conversation and this being interpreted to the clinician as 'He says "no" '.

4 *Substitution* – occurs where the interpreter replaces what has been said by something which has not been said. It may be difficult to

believe that this happens, and it may also be tempting to be very angry with interpreters who do this, but in fact every social conversation we have involves our making assumptions about other people, and interpreters are just acting on a process that happens in discussions anyway.

5   *Role exchange* – occurs when the interpreter takes over the role of interviewer and substitutes the interviewer's questions with those of his own. Problems in this area will of course depend on the nature of the role the clinician and the interpreter believe the interpreter should have – if the clinician's model for correct interpreter practice differs from that of the interpreter, there will almost inevitably be role problems.

The Vasquez and Javier (1991) scheme for understanding errors is a useful one, but it is lopsided in two crucial respects. Their article is entitled 'The problem with interpreters', and though they do devote time in their study to errors made by interviewers, they follow many others in implying that the primary difficulty is with the interpreter's lack of competence or training. Other studies have consistently highlighted the fact that the often unclear position of interpreters in hospital hierarchies, and the lack of training and sensitivity on the part of interviewers themselves may be crucially important in contributing to failure of interviews with interpreters (Crawford, 1994; Drennan, 1996a, 1996b, in press). In considering what good interpreter practice should be, we need to think not only of the interpreter's skills, but also those of the clinician, and of the functioning of the institution and system in which the interview occurs (Muller, 1994).

The second factor which is given insufficient attention by authors such as Vasquez and Javier (1991) and Marcos (1979) is that there is not necessarily one single correct translation for every word (Muller, 1994). For example, Drennan et al. (1991) document the difficulties with translating the concept of 'sadness' to and from Xhosa, and Muller (1994) notes that the Xhosa word *ukukhathazeka* can mean in English, amongst other things, 'upset', 'hurt', 'heartsore', 'sad', 'grief-stricken', and 'worried'. A good interpreted interview, therefore, will be one which takes due account of the impossibility of finding a perfect translation – what is needed is a method of interpreting which serves the clinical purpose as well as it can.

Suggestions for improving interpreted interviews

Interpreted interviews are difficult – for the interviewer, the client, and the interpreter. They take a long time, and can be awkward to manage socially. The first job of the interviewer and the interpreter is to recognize the difficulties, to anticipate them, and to realize that any interpreted interview represents a less than ideal situation. This does not imply that low standards are acceptable, or that parties should feel hopeless. Instead, it represents a realistic basis on which to build the best possible interview.

Preparation

An interview in which the interpreter and the interviewer have different understandings of their roles and of the goals of the interview cannot flow smoothly. These issues must be discussed, as must details of how long the interview will take, and how issues will be dealt with as they arise. Ideally, the interviewer and the interpreter will have an ongoing, mutually respectful relationship. Even where the interpreter and the interviewer have just met prior to the interview it is best for them to discuss briefly how they plan to work. Interpreters who have little or no experience in the mental health field often need to be reminded that rules of politeness are often broken in mental health interviews – questions and answers about intimate matters, including sexual matters, may be asked. The interpreter may need to convey material which is stated in a crude way – though this may embarrass the interpreter, it may be central to the assessment.

The issue of note-taking should be discussed. Will the interviewer be taking notes? Will the interpreter be taking notes? It may be uncomfortable for a client to have to deal with two people both taking notes. On the other hand, brief notes taken by the interpreter may be very useful clinically. This may be especially important in comments about nonverbal behaviour. Nonverbal behaviour can tell us a great deal about how people feel, and interviewers not conversant with the language of a client are also often unaware of the rules for nonverbal behaviour in that client's culture.

Fatigue is often a major problem in interpreted interviews. This may occur, first, because interpreted interviews are by nature slow and repetitive and, second, because clients may also be unfamiliar and uncomfortable with a style of interview which depends on many questions and answers (Gillis et al., 1982). The interpreter and interviewer need to know in advance whether the interview can be stopped for a break for a few minutes or even resumed on another occasion. They need to plan who may make this judgement and how it may be negotiated amongst the client, the interviewer, and the interpreter.

In preparing for the interview, the clinician is often the person who has more power in the mental health system than the interpreter. It may therefore be relatively difficult for the interpreter to assert his or her views, but both the clinician and the interpreter need to create an atmosphere in which the interpreter can speak freely.

Introducing the interview

On entering the interpreted interview, the client may well be in a situation he or she has not been prepared for. As with any interview, courtesy and respect require the purpose and manner of the interview to be explained, with the added explanation about the presence and role of the interpreter. Depending on the interpreter/interviewer relationship and the roles they have agreed upon, much of the introduction can be done by the interpreter in the home language of the client. This method assumes that the interpreter is competent to undertake this task, and will inform the interviewer if the client begins to discuss matters relevant to the interview. It is important that the client be given the opportunity to comment on and ask questions about the interview process. In cases of patients who are seriously mentally ill, there may be questions about their competence to agree to an interpreted interview, and power relationships make it difficult for any client to refuse an interpreted interview. As much room as possible, however, must be given to the client to understand and comment on the interview format. Framing the beginning of the session in this manner is helpful simply from a practical point of view – the staff involved are less likely to become involved in conflict with the client later in the interview, and if the interpreter and interviewer need to stop and confer about something, it is easier to explain this if the preparatory work has been done.

Many clients, and with good reason, will have concerns about confidentiality in the interview. They may have anticipated talking to one clinician and now they are confronted with two. It is necessary to be clear with the clients exactly how confidentiality will be protected, and how the interviewer and the interpreter fit into an organizational structure which protects confidentiality.

Conducting the interview

Depending on one's views on the role of the interpreter, there will be different rules as to how to conduct the interview. Many people who are involved in training interpreters, for example, insist that the interviewer never ask third-person questions about the client. Instead of asking the interpreter 'Ask her how she came to be in hospital', the interviewer should face the patient and ask directly, 'How did you come to be in hospital?' Addressing the client in the second person, instead of talking in the third person, is thought to be more respectful and to increase rapport. In practice, though, and especially if the interpreter is working as a co-clinician, this may be difficult to sustain consistently.

It is, however, essential to continue the interview with due regard for the client's feelings, and it may be necessary at various points to clarify to the client how the process is working. This would be done anyway in a good mental health interview, but is especially important in an interpreted interview. The sense of intimacy that often develops in an interview without an interpreter is much more difficult to achieve in the interpreted interview and may, in fact, be impossible. It is also difficult in the interpreted interview to create the same level of informality possible in a direct interview. This is another reason why it may be helpful to rely more on comments about the interview process than would be the case in the non-interpreted interview.

This discussion raises a question which has importance in the planning of the interview as well. What are the limits of what can be achieved in an interpreted interview? Is in-depth psychotherapy possible, for example? An answer cannot be given in the abstract, as what can be achieved depends on a number of factors, including the skills, resources, and availability of both the interviewer and the interpreter, the needs and resources of the client, and the resources of the institution or mental health facility. In general, though, it is true to say that it is far more difficult to achieve complex goals in an interpreted interview than in a direct interview, and this needs to be taken into account both in setting goals for the interview and in the way the interview is conducted. During the course of the interview, both interviewer and interpreter need to have a model of their most modest goals for the session, and they should focus on achieving these rather than trying to gain a great deal of detailed information on one small aspect of the client's experience and needs. This does not mean that what is important to the client must be left out – on the contrary, a well-conducted interpreted interview will focus precisely on these central needs but cannot afford the extras which may be possible to gather quite easily in a direct interview.

As mentioned before, fatigue, frustration, and irritation are common reactions to the interpreted interview, and these are often best dealt with if, as they arise, they are discussed sympathetically and openly with the client. Breaks and rescheduling of part of the interview should always be considered, taking into account whether these are possible both for the client and the mental health service providers.

There are, in summary, no hard and fast rules which can be applied to interpreted interviews, and rigid guidelines cannot anticipate all possibilities for the interview. A good interpreted interview, though, should show all the features of an excellent direct interview, with careful attention to how the process is working and the influence of this process on all parties, and especially on the client.

Discussions after the interview

If at all possible, time should be scheduled immediately after the interview for the interpreter and interviewer to discuss the interview. This is especially helpful where assessments need to be made of the client's mood during the interview, the client's cognitive state, and the form versus content of language used by the client. It is useful if verbatim examples (in the client's home language) of aspects of the client's speech can be recorded.

This post-interview discussion will depend for its success not only on how competent the interpreter and the interviewer are, but also on the quality of their relationship and how free each feels to speak in front of the other. If the interviewer has a higher status than the interpreter (as is often the case), the interpreter may be anxious not to appear inadequate to a higher-status person, and the interviewer, conversely, may be afraid of losing the interpreter's respect if the interviewer does not know more than the interpreter. These concerns about status, though understandable and almost always present, can block open talk about the interview. If an atmosphere of mutual respect and trust can be built up in which it is permissible for both parties to speculate about what has happened without worrying too soon whether the speculations are right, then ideas can flow back and forth. If this atmosphere of debate is successful, then the client will have the benefit of two people's discussion about whatever the client's needs are – and may, in this respect, be getting a better service than someone interviewed directly. This is a difficult but worthwhile goal to strive for.

Having spent much of this chapter dealing with the specifics of interpreting, we now turn briefly to broader issues in thinking about language diversity in mental health care.

Taking on the challenge of language diversity in mental health care

As was mentioned early in this chapter, the ideal situation for every mental health interaction is one in which there is no need for an interpreter. Given the reality of the need for interpreters internationally, however, it has been useful to look closely at the interpreter situation. Thinking about interpreting, furthermore, may help us think more clearly about more general issues concerning language and mental health services.

This chapter is not concerned primarily with policy questions (these will be dealt with briefly in Chapter 11), and readers interested in a detailed consideration of language and mental health policy in South Africa are referred to Swartz et al. (1997). Some basic issues in this field will, however, now be considered.

Infrastructural considerations

Wherever mental health services are to be offered in a multilingual society, due care should be given to how easy it is for speakers of different languages to access the services. Are all signs on and within the building (or on the mobile van, etc.) in all the major languages spoken in that area? Are all brochures and information sheets in all the languages? If there are high levels of illiteracy, has this been taken into account, for example, in the use of pictograms on signposts?

Who is the first point of contact for the clients? Even if a multilingual service of good quality is offered, clients may have difficulty dealing with a monolingual and unsympathetic receptionist. Reception and telephone staff need to be prepared for a diverse client population, and even when they cannot speak directly with clients they should know whom they can call to assist if they cannot speak with clients. This first point of contact is often ignored, but it gives the client the first impression of the service.

Entry requirements and clinician competencies

Who should be permitted to practise as mental health workers? Should language proficiency be an entry requirement for training? This should be considered in any training system, as is currently the case at a number of institutions (Swartz & Maw, 1996). Within any training course, in addition, instruction should be given in how to work sensitively in a multilingual context, and in how to work with interpreters.

Specific projects

There have been many interesting projects dealing with language issues in mental health care. At the University of Cape Town, for example, the Bicultural Workers' Project has been designed to provide Xhosa-speaking undergraduates with experience of working as interpreters (Swartz & Maw, 1996). This programme meets service needs and also helps to mentor Xhosa-speaking undergraduates with the hope that some of them will train as clinical psychologists. An important feature of this programme is that it has given educators some insight into the experiences of black students entering an institutional and professional world still dominated by whites (Bass, 1996) This information is very useful in a number of ways – not the least of which is in understanding the experiences of black clients entering a mental health system dominated by whites.

Thinking about the organization of mental health work

Implicit in much of this chapter has been a consideration of how language issues raise questions about the way mental health workers work together. For example, should a very competent professional nurse act as an interpreter for a psychologist, or should the workload be reorganized so that the professional nurse takes sole professional responsibility for the work? Could the upgrading of the clinical skills of multilingual members of mental health teams and the institution of consultation relationships within the team deal with language issues more effectively than focusing on interpreting? Questions such as this are dealt with in more detail by Swartz et al. (1997), and they also raise issues about interprofessional relationships in mental health care – an issue returned to in later chapters. Thinking about multilingualism, though, can also help us think about what happens in mental health work even when the languages spoken by the clinician and the client are ostensibly the same, as we shall see in the next section.

Speaking the same language? Discourses and mental health care

I was once working in a large psychiatric institution where many of the patients were seen by the staff as suffering from schizophrenia. The patients themselves, however, were far more likely to describe themselves as suffering from depression. Shortly after this I moved to a unit where many of the patients, to the staff, were indeed suffering from depression. Some of these patients, however, described themselves as suffering from schizophrenia.

Part of what was happening in these different contexts was that different explanatory models were operating (see Chapter 1). There was good reason for the patients in the psychiatric institution to label themselves as depressed, as they knew depression is less stigmatized and has a better prognosis than schizophrenia. Conversely, the depressed patients had correctly divined that the staff on their unit were fascinated by serious mental disorder and were likely to give more attention to patients they regarded as severely disturbed – hence the attractiveness of the schizophrenia label.

This small example highlights the fact that even when the same words are used by clients and staff, the terms may have different meanings for them. Language diversity occurs not only across languages but also across usages within the same language. The term 'discourse' can have many meanings, and discourse theory is a large and diverse field, but it is useful here to use the term to refer to different ways in which language is used by different groups. Language usage may differ across many different divides, and there may be different discourses for different social and racial groups, different ages and classes, the different genders. In thinking culturally about mental health and illness we need to be sensitive to the fact that usages – both in terms of vocabulary and in terms of sentence construction – may have different meanings for different speech communities. While this is obvious when the languages spoken are different, this is not always so clear when the same language is used in different ways.

One of the most poignant ways in which this can affect mental health care is shown by Kleinman (1988: 77-94), who describes the initial psychiatric care given to a highly successful physician in North America. This physician, a successful white male medical professional, ostensibly comes from the same speech community as the caring and highly competent psychiatrist caring for him. But Kleinman is able to show how the words spoken by the physician-patient are transformed into professional psychiatric discourse by the psychiatrist, and part of the personal experience of illness is lost in the process.

Barrett (1988) has shown how note-taking by mental health professionals structures the way patients are interacted with and viewed, and others have explored the ways in which ward rounds or case conferences about patients can have similar effects (Arluke, 1980; Frader & Bosk, 1981; Swartz, 1992). What these studies underline is that language issues are everywhere – even when the same language is being spoken. One of the enormous advantages of working cross-culturally is that it helps us to see more clearly what the issues are even within our own professional culture. As was noted in Chapter 1, the work of understanding culture and mental health and illness is as much about understanding ourselves as people and professionals as it is about understanding people who appear to be different from us.

Translation of research and clinical instruments

Up to now, I have focused in this chapter on the *interpreting* situation – in which there is a clinician and a client who do not speak the same language. In mental health research and practice, however, there are many situations in which we wish to use instruments such as structured interviews and questionnaires, and to *translate* these into a variety of languages. The translation enterprise may well be as complicated politically and interpersonally as interpretation can be (Drennan et al., 1991), and the issue of translation of psychiatric instruments raises many issues about universalism and cultural relevance, some of which will be considered further in Chapter 3. Technically, though, there are some useful techniques to obtain the best possible translation of an instrument.

Brislin (1986) suggests a number of translation methods. The first of these, *back-translation*, starts translation of the instrument from the source language into the target language. A second translator unfamiliar with the original instrument then translates the translated instrument back into the source language. The original version of the instrument and the back-translated version can be compared, and adjustments to the translation made until the final back-translated version is conceptually the same as the original version.

Brislin (1986) emphasizes the need for *conceptual* as opposed to *linguistic* equivalence in source and translated versions of the instrument. Conceptual equivalence involves equivalence of the instrument in terms of the meaning of the items, rather than in terms of the wording of the items. For example, an inventory developed in the USA to assess depression, such as the Beck Depression Inventory (Beck et al., 1979), may contain the word 'blue' – an American expression for 'sad'. Any translated version of the inventory should convey the conceptual meaning of sadness rather than the literal or linguistic meaning of the colour blue.

Another way of developing translated instruments suggested by Brislin (1986) is the *bilingual* approach. In this method, bilingual people take versions of the instrument in both source and target language, and their responses, which should be consistent across the two language versions, are compared. In this way accuracy of translation can be checked.

Brislin (1986) suggests that it may also be useful to have a *committee* to discuss aspects of the translated instrument. In practice, this may form a very useful adjunct to back-translation. It is useful after some rounds of back-translation to call together the various translators and back-translators and to have them discuss contentious aspects of the translation.

As Muller (1994) makes clear, there is no single correct translation of any instrument. There will always be differences in opinion about what is involved conceptually in an instrument, both in the source and target languages. What is important, however, is that the purpose for which the instrument will be used is borne in mind, and that there is agreement amongst those who will actually be using the instrument that it is meaningful and phrased in such a way that it will be as easy and as 'natural' as possible to use.

Translating instruments for research purposes can take literally years of work, if the work is to be done thoroughly. Too often, insufficient consideration is given to this fact. Once again, an empiricist view of language may lead one to expect that translation is simply a matter of finding the right labels for reified things – the process is in fact much more complex.

In this chapter we have looked at some of the complicated and challenging issues raised by linguistic diversity in mental health work. These issues inform and are informed by the ways in which we conduct our business as both practitioners and researchers in the mental health field, and in the next chapter we will look more closely at some of the ways various kinds of practitioners and researchers develop and use their tools.

3
Tools of the trades

How do healers in different systems make sense of
  mental health and illness?
Are diagnostic processes similar across cultures?
What tools do researchers use to undertake
  comparative research, and how do these tools
  take account of cultural differences?

These are some of the questions we will be addressing in this chapter.
Many people who have practised in the mental health field have had
the experience of a client's being diagnosed differently by different
diagnostic systems. For example, the same person could be called
schizophrenic by biomedicine, be seen as bewitched in an African
indigenous healing system, and be viewed as possessed by the devil by
a Pentecostal church (Spiro, 1991). Our job in this chapter will be, first,
to gain some idea of how diagnostic decisions are made in different
healing systems, and then to gain an overview of the use of standard
Western diagnostic instruments and epidemiology in the cross-cultural context. Some of the important questions about how this process
works have already been raised in the discussion of language in
Chapter 2; and language and translation issues are central to the entire
field.

   In keeping with the emphasis in this book on seeing biomedicine as
a cultural product as much as any other system, we shall begin by
exploring diagnosis within Western psychiatry.

Diagnosing mental disorder within Western medicine

Normal and abnormal

How does a Western psychiatrist know that a person is mentally ill? He or she uses standard diagnostic methods, which are themselves dependent on assumptions about normality and abnormality.

Western psychiatry is a branch of biomedicine, within which diagnoses are ideally assumed to relate directly to underlying physical pathology. In the ideal biomedical diagnosis, it should be possible to gather a specific set of signs and symptoms which are unequivocal indicators of an underlying disease. These signs and symptoms, in the ideal world, are unique to a specific disease – other configurations of signs and symptoms will be indicative of another disease (it is recognized in major diagnostic texts that, in fact, this ideal is not attainable – see, for example, DSM-IV, 1994). A 'sign' is anything that can be observed about a patient which may be indicative of disease – such as a swelling, blotches, or results of laboratory examinations. A 'symptom' is what the patient may complain of – pain, tiredness, shortness of breath, for example. The first way, then, that a decision could be made about a diagnosis in biomedicine is on the basis of the assumption of *underlying medical pathology*. Correct treatment in this model consists of treating the underlying pathology and hence eradicating the signs and symptoms – and in this, biomedicine has been spectacularly successful. A further feature of decision-making about mental disorder in the biomedical system is that biomedicine depends on Cartesian dualism (from Descartes in the seventeenth century) – the idea that the mind is separate from the body (Gordon, 1988).

A second tradition in Western decision-making about normality and abnormality relates closely to the medical model described above. In the *psychoanalytic* tradition started by Freud, psychological signs and symptoms, as well as a range of other non-pathological phenomena such as slips of the tongue, relate to underlying pathology of a psychological rather than of a physical nature (Freud, in fact, on various occasions, speculated that with increasing medical sophistication the physical basis of many disorders would be discovered). In this model, the underlying pathology, which may relate to early childhood experiences, is psychic in nature but operates in a manner analogous to physical pathology: it is the cause of the signs and symptoms, and the treatment for the signs and symptoms involves treatment of the underlying pathology. Much has been written about the moral, philosophical, and cultural underpinnings of the Freudian world-view, but for the purposes of the present discussion it is enough to note the similarities structurally between the psychoanalytic system and the medical one. One important contribution of the Freudian tradition, though, is that Freud insisted on there being a range of behaviours in the way people conduct their lives, and refused simply to label behaviour as abnormal. He stressed the continuities between normal and abnormal behaviour, arguing that even well-functioning people live with pathological parts of themselves. He described, for example, the 'polymorphously perverse disposition' (Freud, 1991/1905: 109) of *all* children with respect to sexuality.

This idea of a range of behaviours relates well to the *statistical* view of abnormality. The word 'abnormal' simply means 'different from the norm or rule'. Statistically, it can be argued, there are great variations in human characteristics. Those people who deviate further than most from the norm, or the average, we call 'abnormal'. We can even, in this model, specify how far from average we would want a characteristic to be from the average before we label it abnormal. For example, we may decide to call a man abnormally tall only if he is taller than 95 per cent of other men, say, or 99 per cent, or 99.9 per cent, and so on, depending on our criteria. In the statistical model (theoretically at least), there is no value attached to the term 'abnormal' – it simply means different from most other people, and does not specify in which direction the difference occurs. It would therefore be as accurate to say that an exceptionally intelligent person is as abnormal intellectually as someone with what the American Psychiatric Association would term mental retardation (DSM-IV, 1994).

Clinicians, though, are usually more interested in diagnosing people who have problems in living rather than those who do very well (though much may be learned from those who do well), so there is often added to the statistical definition a component dealing with *impairment of functioning.* This may relate to difficulties with intimate relationships, with social functioning and social role, and with work and learning tasks, for example.

All these views, in various ways, influence the way that psychiatric diagnoses are currently made. They have in common two key features: they do not make reference to spiritual or supernatural causation of abnormality, and they do not, on the surface, make moral judgements about abnormality. Abnormality is viewed as a medical or psychological problem, or as evidence of difference from the norm. The extent to which these models of abnormality do, in fact, avoid moral judgements can be hotly debated (Gordon, 1988; Lock, 1987). The important point, though, is that the scientific attitude adopted in these approaches emphasizes rationality and a dispassionate approach rather than a moralistic one.

What is a psychiatric diagnosis?

The most obvious use of diagnosis is to provide the clinician with a picture of what is happening with the patient, and then to develop a treatment plan. Diagnosis is also necessary so that professionals can easily communicate with one another about patients and pool clinical and research findings.

The critical psychiatry and anti-psychiatry traditions (Ingleby, 1981; Laing, 1960; Szasz, 1961, 1971), which had their heyday in the 1960s and 1970s, drew attention to some of the more sinister uses to which diagnosis could be put. People who are abnormal, in the sense of not fitting in with current social norms, can be diagnosed and labelled as ill – Littlewood and Lipsedge's (1989) recall of 'drapetomania' as mentioned in Chapter 1 exemplifies this problem. In this way, psychiatric diagnoses can become instruments of social control. Behaviour unacceptable to society can be labelled and then seen as needing treatment or eradication. There is no question that medical metaphors and metaphors of hygiene were extensively used during the Nazi regime (Lifton, 1986). Jews, gypsies, homosexuals, and others were seen as symptomatic of a social illness that needed to be eradicated. Similarly, in the USSR psychiatry, and psychiatric diagnosis specifically, has been used to deal with political dissidence (Merskey & Shafran, 1986). Though these are extreme examples, they raise general questions about the social and cultural role of the mental health industry and of diagnosis in particular. Psychiatric labelling can be seen as part of a more pervasive social process of *medicalization* whereby social problems are conceived of in medical terms. The solutions, similarly, are conceived of in an individualistic way. Some of these issues will be returned to when we discuss 'stress' as a category, in Chapter 8.

At worst, the anti-psychiatry arguments about psychiatric diagnosis can be unfair in disregarding both the positive achievements of the Western mental health system and the commitment of very many practitioners to the welfare of their clients. An important implication of these arguments, though, is that we need at all times to raise questions about the broader social function of diagnosing people. Diagnoses are not only for helping individual clinicians deal with individual clients but also for establishing and maintaining broad social patterns of relationships between different groups of people. It is possible to show that some diagnoses are used more commonly with some race groups than with others, even where the symptoms are ostensibly the same (Littlewood, 1988; Swartz, 1989, 1991). Similar arguments have been made with respect to gender, and there is evidence that certain diagnoses are associated with either the male or the female gender (Seeman, 1995). For example, women are more consistently labelled as having unipolar depression than are men (Shaw et al., 1995), and in persons with substance abuse disorders, men are far more likely to also receive the diagnosis of antisocial personality disorder (Lex, 1995).

By this stage, it should be clear that a psychiatric diagnosis is not simply a label for a set of signs and symptoms which exist 'out there', but a social act which reinforces social relationships (such as those between diagnoser and diagnosed, and between the sick and healthy). Kleinman (1988:7) argues that diagnosis is an *interpretation* of someone's experience. This view is in keeping with the hermeneutic approach we have discussed in the previous two chapters.

The important feature of all the above observations about psychiatric diagnosis is that although the process follows strict rules and is underpinned by much research, it remains part of a cultural system of interacting with and making meaning in the world. Psychiatric diagnosis involves extracting from a person's story only certain pieces of information – those which form pieces to complete a diagnostic puzzle. This statement does nothing to detract from the value and benefits of psychiatric diagnosis, but it reminds us that a psychiatric diagnosis represents one very particular way of interpreting someone's experience. It leaves out other aspects of the person. Similarly, within Western medicine diagnoses are based on an individualistic view of the person, and attempt to exclude spiritual and religious beliefs from diagnosis.

Culture and the DSM-IV

The *Diagnostic and statistical manual of mental disorders* (Fourth Edition), or DSM-IV, was published by the American Psychiatric Association in 1994. The DSM-IV is one of the most widely-used diagnostic systems in the world, along with the *ICD-10 classification of mental and behavioural disorders* (ICD-10), published by the World Health Organization in 1992. The dominance of these systems reflects the dominance of European and North American psychiatry internationally, but they are by no means the only systems (Lee, 1996a). The two systems share many characteristics (though there are also important differences), but given the widespread use of the DSM-IV in southern Africa, the DSM-IV will form the focus of this section. The DSM-IV represents a further version of the tradition started in 1980 with the publication of the DSM-III. Although there had been two previous editions of the DSM, starting in 1952, the DSM-III marked a major consolidation of an empirical, research-based approach to classification in American psychiatry.

It is useful in introducing the DSM-IV to consider some of the basic principles which underpinned the DSM-III, and which were carried over into the new edition. The aims in the design of the DSM-III included:

- clinical usefulness for making treatment and management decisions in varied clinical settings

- reliability of diagnostic categories
- acceptability to clinicians and researchers of various theoretical orientations (APA, 1980: 2)

The DSM-III was designed, therefore, so that it could be widely used in a standard way by a variety of people with a variety of perspectives on mental disorder. This is in keeping both with universalism and with an attempt to make a classification system which, as far as possible, is empiricist in its approach – depending on the collection of observable symptoms and avoiding reliance on any specific theory of aetiology (the technical term for causation of disease).

> For most of the DSM-III disorders ... the etiology is unknown ... The approach taken in DSM-III is atheoretical with regard to etiology or pathophysiological process except for those disorders for which this is well established and therefore included in the definition of the disorder. (APA, 1980: 6-7)

Even the term 'neurotic disorder' in the DSM-III, which comes historically from psychoanalysis, is used simply descriptively. The insistence in the DSM-III on being atheoretical and descriptive does, in fact, derive from a particular theoretical perspective – that of empiricism. As we have seen, other views of language would argue that it is not possible to use a descriptive term without being involved in some form of interpretive or hermeneutic exercise.

An important consequence of this empirical approach is that the DSM-III is involved only in the labelling of a group of symptoms, and not in the labelling of a whole person. Like previous classificatory systems, the DSM-III explicitly rejects the idea that there can be a person who is 'a schizophrenic', for example (APA, 1980; Wing et al., 1974). Instead, the person is called 'a person with schizophrenia' – the disorder does not define the whole person.

Social and cultural factors are accounted for to some degree in the DSM-III by the multiaxial system. In this system, five axes are used to diagnose in each case:

AXIS 1 Clinical Syndromes
AXIS 2 Personality Disorders
        Specific Developmental Disorders
AXIS 3 Physical Disorders and Conditions
AXIS 4 Severity of Psychosocial Stressors
AXIS 5 Highest Level of Adaptive Functioning Past Year
        (APA, 1980: 23)

It is not necessary here to explain how the multiaxial system works, but it is clear that the last two axes are both concerned with factors in the social environment which impact on a person's functioning and on how others expect the person to behave.

Following extensive criticism of the DSM-III for its universalist stance, which gave relatively little attention to cultural factors, the DSM-IV pays much more attention to cultural factors. International advisers were called in to 'ensure cultural sensitivity, applicability for international mental health professionals, and greater compatibility with ICD-10' (DSM-IV, 1994: 864). Most of these advisers, though, were located either in Europe or North America, with three of the 182 advisers coming from sub-Saharan African countries. There were also 64 advisers on cross-cultural issues, again mainly North American based, but with a vast range of expertise in the fields of cross-cultural psychiatry and medical anthropology internationally.

Introducing the book based on the deliberations of the Conference on Culture and Psychiatric Diagnosis, Eisenberg (1996) notes:

> Taking culture into account is not simply an issue of whether it is legitimate to apply mainstream schemata to people from other cultures. Diagnosis itself is a cultural issue in mainstream society. (Eisenberg, 1996: xiii)

This comment sets the tone for a remarkable collection of papers, all of which try to wrestle with the question of the extent to which DSM-IV diagnoses, and the DSM-IV enterprise itself, can begin to deal with a diverse world (Mezzich et al., 1996). What makes the collection especially remarkable is the fact that many of the contributors to the volume are hermeneutically-oriented in their thinking and well aware of the culture-boundedness of the DSM-IV. Yet they attempt to engage with the reality of the DSM-IV in order to produce an approach which will be of help to a wide range of patients.

Perhaps inevitably, the attempts made by this group to influence the construction of the DSM-IV were not as far-reaching as some had hoped (Good, 1996: 127), though there were significant advances on DSM-III. One important achievement is that cultural factors are considered throughout the DSM-IV, and not just added as an after-thought. Attempts, however, to change the approach to the DSM-IV in the light of cross-cultural evidence were not fully realized:

> The primary thrust and philosophic commitments of the DSM-IV remained largely impervious to the empirical and ultimately political claims of those at the cultural margins of American society. (Good, 1996: 128)

It is precisely these North American 'margins' that we in southern Africa are chiefly engaged with. Our society does not look like the mainstream American society that created the DSM-IV, and it is a matter of international politics that we should be trying at times to fit our patients and ourselves unthinkingly into this foreign mould.

Good notes further the importance of a commitment to 'a view of psychopathology as social and cultural' (Good, 1996: 129). This does not deny the role of biology in mental disorder, but emphasizes those dimensions which the DSM-IV tends to ignore or take for granted. The politics involved in relegating the proposals on cultural formulation to half of an appendix in the final DSM-IV are outlined by Lewis-Fernández (1996a). An important consequence of the proposals, though, is that the journal *Culture, Medicine and Psychiatry* has begun publishing a series of clinical case reports which provide evidence for the utility of the cultural formulation model (outlined briefly below), and for thinking broadly about cultural factors in diagnostic decision-making (Fleming, 1996; Lewis-Fernández, 1996b; Lim & Lin, 1996). Cases such as these, which will be appearing regularly in the journal, provide an interesting model.

What, though, has appeared in the DSM-IV itself with respect to cultural issues? In introducing 'ethnic and cultural considerations', the DSM-IV argues:

> A clinician who is unfamiliar with the nuances of an individual's frame of reference may incorrectly judge as psychopathology those normal variations in behavior, belief, or experience that are particular to the individual's culture. For example, certain religious practices or beliefs (for example, hearing or seeing a deceased relative during bereavement) may be misdiagnosed as manifestations of a Psychotic Disorder. Applying Personality Disorder criteria across cultural settings may be especially difficult because of the wide cultural variation in concepts of self, styles of communication, and coping mechanisms. (DSM-IV, 1994: xxiv)

The DSM-IV continues, arguing that 'the international acceptance of the DSM suggests that this classification is useful in describing mental disorders *as they are experienced* by individuals throughout the world' (DSM-IV, 1994: xxiv, emphasis added), but adds that 'the symptoms and course of a number of DSM-IV disorders are influenced by cultural and ethnic factors' (DSM-IV, 1994: xxiv). Through these statements some basic assumptions of the DSM-IV system with respect to culture are made clear. First, there seems to be no distinction made between symptoms as they are diagnosed or reported by a clinician (disease) and symptoms as they are experienced in a range of settings (illness). In addition, there is the clear idea that the DSM categories represent, in general, an underlying universal, which may be present and progress differently in different contexts (cf. Good, 1996).

The DSM-IV makes three categories of provision for cultural and ethnic factors in diagnosis. First, it mentions cultural differences as they affect particular disorders mentioned in the body of the DSM-IV text; second, it provides an appendix which discusses how to include consideration of cultural factors in decision-making about clients and, in the same appendix, includes a glossary of culture-bound syndromes (DSM-IV, 1994: 843-849). What the DSM-IV terms the 'cultural formulation' of the patient, which supplements the multiaxial classification, considers:

- cultural identity of the individual
- cultural explanations of the individual's illness
- cultural factors related to psychosocial environment and level of functioning
- cultural elements of the relationship between the individual and the clinician
- overall cultural assessment for diagnosis and care (DSM-IV, 1994: 843-844)

This practical and useful guideline to culture-sensitive assessment within the Western universalist system (and the model for the cultural formulation series in *Culture, Medicine and Psychiatry*) is supplemented with the most extensively-studied culture-bound syndromes existing outside the DSM-IV parameters. As we will see when we consider culture-bound syndromes in Chapter 7, there is debate as to what is the most useful definition of culture-bound syndromes, and it is not entirely clear what the relationship should be between use of a culture-bound syndrome label and the rest of the DSM-IV classification system.

In summary, it appears that the DSM-IV, though being primarily a universalist product of North American (and European) psychiatry, has begun a process of recognizing the importance of cultural diversity in mental health work. At this stage, the adaptations to the DSM system as a result of cultural considerations are not fully thought through or integrated into DSM thinking, nor have the challenging issues raised by cultural relativism been taken on. The recognition of cultural factors as important, however, is a significant step, and it will be interesting to see what develops in later versions of the DSM system.

Throughout this section there have been two implicit questions raised about the DSM-IV as a diagnostic instrument. The first of these concerns how the DSM-IV deals with cultural diversity, and has been considered in some detail above. The second concerns the DSM-IV itself as a cultural product. We have seen that the DSM-IV emphasizes certain core values of Western psychiatry and of biomedicine as a whole – such as moral neutrality, faith in science, and reliance on empirical research in advancing knowledge. These values give the DSM-IV much of its strength and vitality. It will be useful, however, to remember these core values for comparative purposes when we consider other diagnostic systems. It is also important to mention that in the actual process of professional socialization into psychiatry (and into biomedicine more generally), there is often, at the same time, a less obvious and less rational system of enculturation into seeing the world in a professional way (Light, 1980). Hunter (1996), in exploring some of the paradoxes of clinical learning, notes the tension between sets of injunctions facing clinicians, such as 'avoid the anecdotal' versus 'pay attention to stories' (p. 231); 'the research shows' versus 'in my experience' (p. 233); and 'medicine as a science' versus 'medicine as an art' (p. 234). In all cases, the DSM-IV emphasizes the rational, replicable aspects of diagnosis, and takes its place alongside current movements in biomedicine, such as the current trend to what is termed evidence-based medicine. But irrationality and clinical folklore also play a part in how diagnostic and clinical skills are learned (Light, 1980; Swartz, 1991a). We will now consider approaches which are more likely to emphasize these aspects in the diagnostic process.

Diagnosing mental illness in Africa

Preliminary issues

To speak of African indigenous healing as though it is a single, unified system is probably even more inaccurate than it is to generalize about the way biomedicine is practised around the world. There is great variety in methods, aims, and theories of illness (Feierman & Janzen, 1992; Peltzer, 1995). There is also a problem in seeing the world as divided neatly in two – the rational, scientific, Western world versus the irrational, spiritual, non-Western world (Boonzaier & Sharp, 1988;

Swartz 1985b). There are a number of romantic ideas about mental disorder in non-Western countries, including the following:

1 mental illness does not exist in developing countries; or
2 mental illness is not recognized as pathological; or
3 where it does exist, it is accepted in an unstigmatized manner; or
4 all mental illnesses are cured by indigenous healers.

All these myths have been shown to be false by epidemiological, anthropological, and other research (Asuni et al., 1994; Binedell, 1993; Desjarlais et al., 1995; Murphy, 1976; Ngubane, 1977; Orley, 1970; Orley & Wing, 1979; Peltzer & Ebigbo, 1989; WHO, 1973, 1979). What is true, by contrast, is that some experiences, which Western psychiatrists have, in the past, incorrectly labelled as mental illness, are acceptable forms of experience in those cultures. These experiences include attribution of misfortune to bewitchment and spirit possession, and the state of emotional upheaval which may precede becoming an indigenous healer (Bührmann, 1977, 1982, 1984; Swartz, 1986, 1987b).

Whereas Western psychiatry, in its presentation of itself as rational and scientific, tends to underplay non-rational aspects in diagnostic practice (Wing, 1978), the reverse has tended to be true for African indigenous healing. This may be more a matter of presentation than of substance, and there have been vigorous arguments to show the similarities between various systems (Boonzaier, 1985). There have also been attempts to show that non-rational or emotional processes in African indigenous healing are similar to the emotional upheaval which may be involved in the process of becoming a Western psychotherapist (Bührmann, 1983a, 1983b, 1984), but the image of Western medicine and psychiatry as rational is far more widely propagated. The authority of Western mental health care rests largely on claims to scientific respectability (it is partly for this reason that the psychoanalytic tradition is not especially powerful at present, as it is best understood through a hermeneutic rather than an empiricist view of science). Much of the authority of African indigenous healing, to those who use it, rests on rather different claims. This is well illustrated by Reynolds (1996) who shows that indigenous healers in

Zimbabwe tend to emphasize the mystical aspects of how they gained their clinical knowledge, but to defocus from the fact that they also learn from direct teaching and observing the work of other healers.

There are political issues at stake in discussing both the similarities and differences between biomedical and African healing systems. In South Africa, apartheid ideology played a role in emphasizing the irrational aspects of indigenous healing, and in arguing that 'naturally' Africans chose this system of healing in preference to Western medicine (Swartz, 1986, 1987b, 1995). This claim implied that African people had a choice about which system of healing to use, when in fact formal health services, and mental health services in particular, were simply not widely available (Centre for the Study of Health Policy, 1990; Freeman, 1989). Furthermore, apart from being inaccurate, the image of the irrational African contrasted with the rational, logical Westerner smacks of racism – the very racism Littlewood and Lipsedge (1997) wish to expose as prevalent in the transcultural psychiatry field. On the other hand, though, in the post-independence African context, a reclaiming of what is to be valued in indigenous healing has been important, and there have also been political gains to be made in asserting both that indigenous healing has a rational basis in many respects, and that it may be relatively difficult for outsiders to understand and evaluate (Last & Chavunduka, 1989; Swartz, 1996). These political issues are complex and strongly affect what is said about culture and mental health in Africa (Swartz, 1995, 1996), but they are not our chief concern here. It is enough to note that they do play an important role in the way we discuss all issues.

Features of African indigenous diagnostic practice

We have seen that three central features of Western diagnostic practice important in the construction of the DSM-IV are: i) the development of a reliable instrument which, as far as possible, should be able to be used globally; ii) a system of diagnosis which focuses ideally on distinctive sets of features and attempts to create a taxonomy (an organized system of categories) without, in most cases, reference to the causes of disorders; and iii) an approach to clinical practice in which a diagnosis precedes and informs the treatment phase. African indigenous healing has different emphases in its approach to these issues, each of which will be considered here.

Reliability of diagnosis

Introducing her book on healing amongst Zulu people, Ngubane (1977) notes the distinction between *umkhuhlane* and *ukufa kwabantu*. The former means illness that 'just happens' (p. 24), such as smallpox or influenza. These illnesses are considered universal and able to be treated biomedically, in a non-ritualized way. *Ukufa kwabantu* ('diseases of the African people'), on the other hand, are specifically African. Although African indigenous healing does make claims in its ability to treat biomedical illnesses, the major focus is on *ukufa kwabantu*. This is exactly the opposite emphasis from the DSM-IV, which concerns itself with creating a universal system, and deals with cultural factors only at the margins of that system.

The interrelationship of this difference in diagnostic practice is profound. First, there is considerable interest in local variation in phenomena, and it is regarded as a diagnostic achievement rather than a diagnostic failure that a phenomenon like *amafufunyana* (a form of spirit possession or hysteria occurring amongst Zulu and Xhosa-speakers – we shall learn more about it in Chapter 7), for example, may have different diagnostic features in different contexts. Second, where Western psychiatry tries to incorporate new phenomena into existing categories, and is cautious about developing new categories, there is not necessarily the same caution in African systems (Kirk, 1996). The heavy reliance on contextual information in making sense of these phenomena – a hermeneutic approach – contrasts with the attempt to make the DSM-IV as context-free as possible. Third, different schools or groups of healers working in different contexts may approach the question of diagnosis in slightly different ways. Part of the reason for this will also be seen in the next two subsections. It is also important to consider the possibility that, as Last (1992) has noted from his fieldwork in Nigeria, patients and their kin do not necessarily expect their traditional doctors to have a consistent theory or form a cohesive group. Instead they accept that the different systems and methods of medicine have only a limited validity, although people do treat traditional medicine also as a residual category when other methods seem too dangerous or simply inadequate. (Last, 1992: 398)

Diagnosis, causation, and symptoms

Some authors have attempted to make organized lists of indigenous illnesses along similar lines to the construction of the DSM-IV (Edwards et al., 1982; cf. Ensink & Robertson, 1996). Though this can be useful, the presentation of indigenous categories as though they are simply groupings of symptoms is potentially misleading. Diagnosis in African indigenous healing may be better understood as related to theories of causation of illness rather than simply to taxonomies. It would be possible, therefore, for two people to receive the same diagnosis (of bewitchment, say), but with quite different symptom patterns. This can, in fact, happen to a degree even with DSM-IV categories, where there may be an overlap in symptom profiles across two patients but marked differences in some aspects of presentation, and it is accepted in the DSM-IV that this occurs, but the ideal is a set of mutually exclusive categories. In African indigenous diagnostic practice, however, large differences in overt symptoms is not necessarily a problem, as what counts is the aetiology or cause. In this respect, the system is far more like psychoanalysis which can link a wide range of behaviour into a single category on the basis of aetiology. For example, in psychoanalysis, excessive neatness and/or excessive untidiness may both be linked to excessive concern with bowel movements.

African ideas about causation of illness relate to a range of issues in the natural, social, personal, spiritual, and political realms. Sinzingre and Zempléni (1992: 315) indicate how closely diagnostic and causation issues are related in African medicine by listing four key questions that need to be asked about any illness. These are: Which sickness is it? How has it happened? Who or what produced it? Why did it occur at this moment in this individual? These questions (which are essentially questions about explanatory models, as discussed in Chapter 1) are linked, so that different illnesses may relate to disruptions in different areas. For example, illness may be related to an ecological imbalance, to pollution, to impaired social relationships, to bewitchment, or sorcery (because of jealousy or for other reasons), or through disturbed relationships with the spiritual world – such as not complying with the wishes of ancestors (Green, 1997; Ngubane, 1977).

Given the fluidity with which African indigenous diagnostic labels can be used, and given the role of theories of cause in these labels, the question arises: are these labels primarily illness or disease labels? If disease is seen to refer only to professional, Western constructions, then the labels cannot be disease labels, by definition. But the question still needs to be asked: to what extent do diagnoses given by indigenous healers correspond to the illness experience of the sufferer? Many authors have a romantic view of how indigenous healers are automatically more in touch with their clients than are Western-trained professionals, but there is no reason why this is necessarily true (Swartz, 1996). Spiro (1991) has shown that amongst African patients, as with patients elsewhere, the family, the patient, and the practitioner may all hold different labels and views as to the cause of illness. It is a mistake to assume therefore that African indigenous healing necessarily reflects the views of its patients, or that patients who use the system may not have differences of opinion with the healers they see (cf. Ensink & Robertson, 1997).

Relationship between diagnosis and treatment

The assessment process in Western psychiatry, as has already been mentioned, is viewed as separate and prior to the treatment phase. Assessment generally involves asking a great many questions – collecting a psychiatric history, and finding out about current mental state and functioning. This tradition of asking many questions of the individual patient is not as strongly emphasized in African indigenous healing. Instead, the healer may make statements to the patient, and whoever else is present, and adapt the interpretations of what is troubling the patient by carefully monitoring the reactions of those around. In psychiatric settings, patients more familiar with this mode of clinical interaction may find the ongoing direct questioning of psychiatric assessment especially difficult to deal with (Gillis et al., 1982; Parry & Swartz, 1997; Swartz et al., 1985).

In African indigenous healing, as in many other forms of healing, the biomedical divisions between assessment and treatment, and between mind and body, are not as rigid. The process of healing itself – which may, for example, involve dance and drumming – will provide more information about the problem as the treatment proceeds (Bührmann, 1981; Turner, 1968). African indigenous healing may share some characteristics with those branches of psychotherapy which emphasize the healing relationship above the diagnostic acumen of the clinician, and which would regard vigorous assessment at the outset of treatment as a potential barrier between therapist and client (see, for example, Holdstock, 1981a, 1981b; Rogers, 1961). It is also important to note that a relative lack of attention to systematization of fine-grained diagnostic decisions may also reflect the social position of healing in a particular society, and the importance given to it in that society. The ways in which diagnostic practices become more or less systematic over time will depend on a variety of social forces (Last, 1992). Over the past thirty years or so, it is probably true to say that the central unifying trend in Western psychiatry has been, for various reasons, a concern with an over-arching taxonomy. This concern has not necessarily been reflected in all healing systems. Every healing system, though, depends for its credibility, at least partly, on its perceived therapeutic or social successes. Treatment concerns, especially where many healers compete for the same clientele, may predominate over diagnostic considerations.

In summary, it is a mistake to view diagnosis in African indigenous healing as the same in all respects as biomedicine. Diagnosis is more fluidly related to both theories of cause and to the treatment process itself. There may be a variety of social and contextual reasons for this, but whatever these are, it is important to bear in mind, in planning any research in the mental health field, that systems of healing differ not only in terms of the actual labels and diagnoses given but also in terms of how diagnostic systems are constructed. This has implications for the practice of epidemiology cross-culturally, and we shall consider epidemiology in the mental health context in the following section.

Epidemiology and mental health in cultural perspective

Epidemiology has been defined as 'the study of the distribution and determinants of health-related states or events in specified populations, and the application of this study to the control of health problems' (Last, 1988, as quoted by Beaglehole et al., 1993: 3). The classic focus of study of epidemiology was, in the past, communicable diseases. In the nineteenth century, John Snow established that cholera in London could be related to contaminated water. This classic study laid the basis for the foundation of modern epidemiology. Currently, epidemiology remains concerned about communicable diseases such as tuberculosis and AIDS, but there is also important work in the area of diseases of lifestyle, such as hypertension and coronary heart disease. Epidemiological studies are also conducted on health-related behavioural phenomena, such as substance abuse and violence. Expertise in the mental health area is essential to epidemiologists studying behavioural and lifestyle phenomena, as well as the epidemiology of mental disorders themselves.

There is much, therefore, that an understanding of mental health issues can offer to epidemiology, and the reader is referred elsewhere for a broader discussion of this (Parry & Swartz, 1997). In this section we shall focus only on some key considerations at the interface between epidemiology and mental health work. As epidemiology is used extensively to describe the distribution and course of mental disorders and distress internationally, and to evaluate intervention programmes, a basic understanding of epidemiology is necessary for anyone reading the literature on culture and mental health.

Some central epidemiological concepts

Case definition

Fundamental to the study of epidemiology is the careful definition and assessment of the condition being studied. If epidemiology is to be able to tell us anything about the distribution of diseases and health-related conditions internationally, we have to be sure that conditions are being described in a valid (accurate) and reliable (replicable) way. We have seen how the DSM-IV (1994) attempts to provide just such a form of definition for the mental health field, but this approach has both limitations and potential problems. Using DSM-IV criteria alone may obscure some of the purpose of the investigation, as criteria may differ from study to study (Wing et al., 1981). For example, a study which tries to document the extent of depression amongst women in a rural village may use different criteria for case definition from a study trying to assess the need for treatment of depressed women in that same village. This is because we know that not all depression needs treatment. Some people who are depressed will get better without any treatment. It is therefore imperative that we think not only of the definition of the symptoms we need for any study, but also of what the study is for.

In a cross-cultural context, some issues of case definition become quite complex (and fascinating). For example, it appears from a number of studies that guilt may be less of a prominent feature of depression in Africa than in Britain or North America (Abas & Broadhead, 1997), and that there may be different ways of experiencing emotions, such as guilt, internationally (Kleinman, 1986; Leff, 1988), which may relate to how societies are organized (Lutz, 1985; Shweder & Bourne, 1982). If we find, then, a resident of New York who is depressed and suffers from feelings of guilt, and we find another person from rural Zambia who reports essentially the same feelings as recordable in a standard (reliable) way, are we in fact talking about the same emotion in both contexts? If guilt is less common, say, in Zambia, is it a more serious condition? This question is empirical in part in the sense that it would be possible to conduct a study to see whether the consequences of the emotion would be different in the two contexts.

But the question is also theoretical – or hermeneutic – in that it raises questions about what our labels mean in different contexts.

Researchers have used a number of techniques to improve the validity of standard case-finding instruments cross-culturally. These include having as members of the research team staff who are familiar with the cultural background of the respondents (Dhadphale & Ellison, 1983; Rumble et al., 1996). Some of the difficulties associated with having a team member act as an expert on the culture of a patient or respondent have been discussed in the previous chapter. Other authors have suggested adding items which have local relevance and meaning to standard instruments (for example, Ebigbo, 1982), or of aiming for conceptual as opposed to linguistic equivalence in the translation of standard instruments (Brislin, 1986). This raises the question of what, once these adaptations have been made, we are actually measuring – an issue which we shall return to when we consider depression cross-culturally in Chapter 5. If we simply apply standard instruments like those derived from the DSM-IV then we shall surely be imposing an inappropriate framework on our data – what Kleinman (1977, 1988) calls a 'category mistake'. But if we change our data-collection procedures, and the instruments themselves, then to what extent are we talking about comparable categories? This issue is not easily solved, but as Kleinman (1986) has shown, it is possible to conduct research which keeps in mind both the need for comparability across studies, and the need to respect local context. There can be no easy formula as to how to conduct good research in this field. It should always be remembered that, though there may be a strong pull simply to use instruments which have been used elsewhere, as these are recognizable and respected internationally, there is no point in conducting research in which there has been invalid case definition.

The concept of causation

Epidemiologists have considered a number of ways in which we can begin to assess whether Condition A causes Outcome B. From a research design point of view, the ideal method of demonstrating cause is by conducting an experiment known as a randomized controlled trial. From a practical, and especially from an ethical, point of view, though, it is often not possible to conduct experiments. For example, if we believe smoking causes lung cancer, we cannot design an experiment in which we make some previously healthy people smoke cigarettes so that we can see how many of them develop lung cancer. Similarly, if we believe that unemployment causes depression, we cannot, for the sake of our research, take away jobs from employed people.

We are instead forced to think generally about what makes causation more likely in a study. Beaglehole et al. (1993) summarize epidemiological guidelines for causation as follows:

Temporal relation	Does the cause precede the effect? (Essential)
Plausibility	Is the association consistent with other knowledge?
Consistency	Have similar results been shown in other studies?
Strength	What is the strength of association between cause and effect?
Dose-response relationship	Is increased exposure to the possible cause associated with increased effect?
Reversibility	Does the removal of a possible cause lead to a reduction of disease risk?
Study design	Is the evidence based on a strong study design?

continued

Judging the evidence	How many lines of evidence lead to the conclusion?

(Abbreviated from Beaglehole et al., 1993: 76)

These guidelines are very useful, especially to the extent that they force us to think carefully about what causes mental illness and distress, and what may simply be associated with it. They also help us to think critically about what we may mean when we suggest that one form of social or cultural organization may be better or worse for mental health than another. It is far too easy to attribute mental ill-health to social arrangements of which we disapprove, without thinking clearly about what criteria we are using to claim causation.

The concept of risk

Epidemiologically, the definition of risk is quite simple. Any person who can potentially contract a condition is at risk for that condition. For example, say we wish to work out which part of the population is at risk for postpartum depression (depression following childbirth). Men are clearly not at risk. Women – but only women who have recently given birth – are at risk. Depending on our definition of post-partum depression, we shall also be able to define precisely what we mean by 'recently' – the DSM-IV (1994: 387) requires the onset to be within four weeks of the birth. It must be remembered, furthermore, that anybody who already has a condition cannot be at risk of contract-ing it – if, for example, a woman is severely depressed prior to and during childbirth, she is not at risk for postpartum depression. She may well continue to be depressed, and her depression may even get worse, but the depression cannot be of postpartum onset.

The concept of risk is central in epidemiology because it is very unusual to be able to find a cause for any health problem which oper-ates in every single case. Not everybody who smokes, for example, contracts lung cancer, and many people with lung cancer have never smoked. We do know, however, that the chances of contracting lung cancer are far greater amongst smokers than amongst non-smokers. This is what we call risk – and the risk can be calculated. We know, for example, that a baby born in Afghanistan is approximately 39 times more likely to die in infancy than a baby born in Japan (calculated from Beagehole, et al., 1993: 23). Epidemiologically, being born in Afghanistan can be seen as a risk factor for infant mortality.

If this use of the term 'risk' seems odd, this is because the epidemiological use of the term is different from how the term is used popularly. Gifford (1986) points out that whereas epidemiologists think statistically, and about populations, clinicians, and people more generally, tend to think of risk as something more personal. Part of the problem we face in trying to apply the lessons of epidemiological research to clinical practice is that people act on the basis of their own experience rather than on the basis of statistics. We know, for example, that a crucial factor in helping people change their sexual behaviour to minimize the risk of HIV infection is whether those people know someone with AIDS. This personal experience of risk is far more powerful than knowledge of the epidemiological facts. Part of the challenge faced by mental health practitioners in the global context is to help personalize and make psychologically real the risks that epidemiological research has shown to affect people (Desjarlais et al., 1995).

The limits of epidemiology

Properly used, epidemiology has much to offer people involved in the cross-cultural study of mental health. To think, however, about psychological states as though they were medical conditions with the same patterns of causation may be problematic (Miller & Swartz, 1992). Epidemiologists may also find it difficult to understand and evaluate the contributions made by small-scale research using ethnographic or other hermeneutic methods (True, 1990). Some of the greatest contributions to the field have been qualitative in nature, and have not fitted easily into the pattern of assessing risk on a broad scale. The true challenge is to take the best from epidemiology and to apply its methods where they are appropriate, but to be aware that there is never one single tool of the trade in the mental health field.

We have seen in this chapter that there are a range of ways of understanding and studying mental health, mental illness, and distress. All of these approaches have their own cultural basis, their own internal logic, and their own strengths and weaknesses. It is our job to evaluate what is useful about any particular approach for a given purpose, and to think about what assumptions underlie any approach – biomedical or other – to understanding mental health and illness. In the next chapter we will explore some ways different types of practitioners work, and the effects of these work settings in the way mental illness is experienced, understood, and treated.

4

Practitioners and their work

WHAT HAPPENS when somebody becomes mentally ill? Some years ago, many mental health practitioners might have answered this question by saying that the person will, if the symptoms are disabling and persistent enough, come to the attention of a mental health professional. Psychiatric services in many countries were organized in keeping with this central idea. There were large psychiatric hospitals in major centres, staffed by a substantial proportion of (and sometimes, in developing countries, all of) the mental health personnel in the country.

Today, the answer might be quite different. Internationally, there has been a trend towards the deinstitutionalization of psychiatric patients (whether and where this has been successful is a topic beyond the scope of this chapter). There has also been increasing emphasis on primary health care and the development of community-based resources for mentally as well as physically ill patients. (We will look more carefully at mental health services in primary health care in a later chapter.) This change might make many practitioners now say that people with mental illness will, in the first instance, come to the attention of the primary health care system.

Though this view is probably more accurate than one which focuses almost exclusively on psychiatric services, it is limited in at least two respects. First, it retains an exclusive focus on the formal biomedical system as a source of help. There are other healing resources – such as indigenous and religious healing – and these are widely used. Second, an important omission is the fact that people also turn for help to members of the public who do not consider themselves part of any healing system at all. Most of us, in times of distress, turn to friends, relatives, or neighbours for help. We may even make use of others who have no formal emotional caring role – such as colleagues at work, people who serve in coffee shops, and so on.

If we are interested in mental health in cultural perspective, it is important that we consider how all sectors of care operate. Kleinman (1980) distinguishes between what he terms the *professional* sector of health care, which in our context includes formal biomedical services, the *folk* sector, which includes indigenous and religious healing, and the *popular* sector, which includes advice from relatives and friends. As we shall see later, the boundaries between these sectors are by no means rigid. It is also true that people make use of all these sectors in different combinations depending on where they feel they can get help. The idea that sophisticated people use only professional services, whereas unsophisticated people feel more at home with folk healing, is not accurate (Boonzaier, 1985). Once we have briefly considered the sectors of healing, we will examine some ways in which people move between them.

Sectors of healing

The professional sector

In much of the world, including southern Africa, the professional sector is almost synonymous with Western biomedicine. This system is by far the most powerful in terms of budgets, degree of organization, and widespread recognition of expertise (Hahn & Gaines, 1985; Lock & Gordon, 1988). Within the biomedical system, psychiatry is the speciality dedicated to understanding and dealing with mental illness. Eisenberg (1995) has shown how the relationships between psychiatry and the social and biological sciences in the USA have changed with changing political circumstances. He emphasizes the role of psychiatry not only as a scientific discipline but also as a social and moral enterprise (Eisenberg, 1988). The history of psychiatry in southern Africa, as in other parts of the colonized world, is intimately linked with the history of colonialism, and with the ensuing political and social history of the region (Swartz, 1986, 1987b; S. Swartz, 1995). Some of this history clearly has to do with ways in which society manages what it perceives as deviance of different kinds. It is interesting that Robben Island, which later achieved notoriety as the place of political imprisonment of such leaders as Nelson Mandela, was at an earlier time used to house 'lunatics', 'lepers', and the 'feeble-minded' (S. Swartz, 1996).

Professions involved in mental health care include psychiatry, clinical psychology, occupational therapy, social work, and psychiatric nursing. The great bulk of professional mental health care, though, especially in lower-income countries, is handled by persons with no necessary special interest in the field – primary care nursing personnel, and general practitioners to a lesser degree. South Africa has a far larger group of professionals specializing in mental health care than do other countries in the region. For example, whereas there are over a thousand clinical psychologists in South Africa, Malawi has (at the time of writing) one indigenous Malawian working as a clinical psychologist. It is also true, though, that there are far fewer mental health professionals for the South African population than in Europe and North America (Freeman, 1989). According to Freeman (1992: 8), the approximate numbers of mental health professionals in South Africa are as follows:

Personnel	Number	Ratio to population
Psychiatrists	290	1: 130 500
Psychologists (total)	2 420	1: 15 200
Clinical psychologists	1 060	1: 35 800
Psychiatric nurses	7 000	1: 5 400
Social workers	7 300	1: 5 200

Freeman (1992: 8) notes further that 'First World ratios are in the region of around 1 psychologist ... and one psychiatrist per 4 000 and 14 000 respectively'. This gives a clear idea of how under-resourced even South Africa is by such standards.

The reasons for there being so many professions involved in mental health care are complex and cannot be gone into here. Within institutional psychiatric care, professionals operate as a multidisciplinary team, with expertise from each profession being used for the greatest good of the patient. In a psychiatric ward, for example, the psychiatrist may prescribe medication; the psychologist involve the patient in individual psychotherapy; the occupational therapist offer social skills training; the psychiatric nurse implement and monitor a ward programme; and the social worker conduct family therapy with the patient's relatives. The idea that there are discrete pockets of information about the way patients function, which can be brought together in the patient's best interests, can be related to two major factors: *i)* historical developments in the increasing specialization of professions in general (Abbott, 1988); and *ii)* the ways that biomedicine conceives of the person as divisible into separable systems for diagnostic and therapeutic purposes (Gordon, 1988; Young, 1980). Interdisciplinary conflicts, overt or hidden, are a common feature of multidisciplinary teams. The conflict relates partly to very different ways of understanding patients, and partly to issues of power and differential remuneration across professions (Miller & Swartz, 1990b, 1991). Some of these issues will be taken up in more detail in Chapter 11.

Over time, and in different contexts, views change as to what the central functions of professionals involved in mental health care are. Before the introduction of antipsychotic medication in the 1950s, much of psychiatric care was primarily custodial – the provision of a place where seriously mentally ill people were segregated from the rest of society. As treatments became more successful, and with the influence of the civil rights movement in the USA in the 1960s, there has been increasing interest in community-based care. Over recent years, the inpatient population of psychiatric institutions across the world has been declining. Psychiatric wards have increasingly opened in general hospitals, and much more care is conducted on an outpatient basis. Deinstitutionalization, though, has led to increasing visibility of the mentally ill to the rest of society, and there is concern about the extent to which psychiatry has abandoned its responsibility to the mentally ill (Mossman, 1997).

The debates about deinstitutionalization cannot be entered into here, but two central points need to be made. First, financial and social realities make it highly unlikely that there will be a return towards institutionalization of the old psychiatric style within the near future. Second, concerns about psychiatry's 'abandonment' of the mentally ill can be understood partly in the light of more general social concerns about the nature of psychiatry as a social institution (Mossman, 1997). There is an enormous tension world-wide between two functions of the mental health system. On the one hand, we expect professional mental health care to be a system which will alleviate and eradicate major social problems. On the other hand, this system functions partly in an administrative manner, processing patients as rapidly as possible through a system of interventions designed in such a way that there will always be enough space for new patients entering the system (Rhodes, 1991; Swartz, 1992). Fabrega (1992:168) distinguishes between what he terms the 'clinical/individualistic' functions of psychiatry and the 'corporate/institutional' functions. He argues that psychiatry is unique as a biomedical speciality 'because its object is still the whole person in all of his or her complexity' (Fabrega, 1992: 169). This makes psychiatry especially vulnerable to conflicts between the clinical and the institutional functions of psychiatry. Rhodes (1991) shows that a central concern in a psychiatric emergency unit in the USA is emptying beds – making space for the arrival of more patients. Core cultural values about psychiatry as a healing discipline are secondary to the administrative pressures of patient load. This phenomenon in many ways is a special case of the more general issue of what Mizrahi (1987) has termed 'getting rid of patients'. This is the necessity, where resources are scarce, to process patients quickly and, therefore, to attend less to their illness experience than might be desirable. This phenomenon is likely to be further reinforced by systems of health care financing which are, of necessity, administered bureaucratically, and which are concerned with limiting professional input as far as possible, in order to contain costs (Eisenberg, 1995).

It is important to take account of social, economic, and political forces influencing the practice of professional mental health care. Without an understanding of these, we may be led to believe that all changes within mental health care are occasioned by professional beliefs about what is best for patients. Clearly, these beliefs are important, but professionals also operate within the context of a broader society which enables and constrains what may be done by them (Kleinman, 1980). One of the myths about professional, as opposed to folk, healing is that it inevitably, and on the basis of empirical science alone, moves towards more effective forms of healing. (See Minde, 1974a – d, 1975a – h, 1976, 1977a – b, for just such a progressivist view of South African mental health services, and Louw, 1986, by contrast, for a far more contextual view of the history of psychology's role in the labour sphere in South Africa.) It is partly, though not entirely, the expectation that biomedicine should be able to operate according to a cultural role for which the financial and infrastructural supports are no longer available (and, in many cases, were never available) that has led to much disillusionment with professional sector services. What is clear is that all sectors of society make extensive use of folk and popular resources, and it is to these that we now turn.

The popular sector

It has been estimated in the USA and in Taiwan that about 70 to 90 per cent of all illness episodes are dealt with within the popular sector (Kleinman, 1980: 50). This sector consists of a network of people, including family members, neighbours, and other social groups, to whom people turn when they become ill. Popular sector supporters and advisers are not formally trained in health care, and often do not consider themselves as having special skills or abilities in this area, but are influential and important. When distressed or ill, we often turn to people around us for help. They may give advice about home treatments for any problem, including diet or lifestyle changes, may suggest the taking of medicines of various kinds (over the counter, herbal, etc.), and may suggest where to go for further help. The question of whether popular sector helpers adequately treat or change the course of illness has not been extensively researched (Helman, 1994: 87).

The popular sector will play a role in helping distressed or ill people, and those around them, decide whether any help from the folk or professional sector is needed, and from whom such help should be sought. Popular perceptions of what is appropriate care will influence the advice given. Cultural and religious factors, as well as previous experiences of healing (positive and negative), will influence the advice given. Other sources of information, such as the media, may also be important here in determining the ways in which the popular sector may operate. Clearly, a key feature of the popular sector is that it is not well organized, and that there will be many different approaches to dealing with illness, not all of them consistent with one another. What was good advice in one generation may be laughed at in the next. This may be partly because older theories are disproved, and partly for more complex reasons of social change.

The popular sector is influenced by and also has an influence on the professional and folk sectors – it is a mistake to see the sectors as completely separate. It is sometimes difficult to track exactly how different influences operate. For example, when a neighbour tells someone she needs treatment for her 'nerves', to what degree can we say that 'nerves' is a popular concept, when there is evidence that it originated within the biomedicine of the last century (Davis, 1989a; Reynolds & Swartz, 1993)? The particular issue of 'nerves' will be taken up again in Chapter 7, but it is not the only example of popular knowledge changing in complex ways in relation to professional and folk knowledge. The area of diet and healthy eating is especially interesting in this regard and, as an example, I shall use some lay knowledge I received as I was growing up. At one time my grandmother believed that any vegetable which grew under the ground (including potatoes and carrots) was fattening, but any vegetable which grew above the ground (such as pumpkin and peas) was not. As professional knowledge about weight control began in the 1960s to target starch as an important source of a fattening diet, potatoes and peas became taboo foods for my grandmother as she claimed they were both starchy, but carrots and pumpkin were not. These changes depended on my grandmother's interpretation of scientific beliefs from her lay perspective. Within the diet industry, claims to scientific respectability are important in influencing lay knowledge – this is part of the reason why what some regarded as the nutritionally bizarre *Beverly Hills diet* (Mazel, 1981) was so spectacularly successful. It had the aura of scientific knowledge about it.

Helman (1994: 87) includes the self-help movement as part of the popular sector. As Helman points out, the key motivation for self-help groups, like other popular sector practices, is that members have *experience* of a certain problem. This experience is valued more highly than education – for example, only a gambler or someone with close personal experience of gambling may join Gamblers' Anonymous. Professional knowledge about gambling is not required, and is not enough for admission. Some self-help groups have, or have had, links with religious organizations – for example, some groups for alcoholics and drug users have Christian links. In practice, there is often a link between self-help groups and professional services – for example, psychiatric institutions may work closely with families of the mentally ill. Information and expertise may flow across professional/popular boundaries. In South Africa, there is increasing emphasis at the level of health policy in obtaining the input of self-help groups, as these groups have an important insider perspective on illness.

Self-help groups may be seen as a special kind of support group (Heller et al., 1984). Support groups are often started by professionals, or by professionals in conjunction with people who have experienced, or are experiencing, the condition the group addresses. In this respect, these groups may span the boundary between the professional and the popular sector. Sometimes popular sector healers who gain expertise may constitute themselves as folk healers in time.

The folk sector

Folk sector healers are people who consider themselves healers by virtue of some special knowledge or quality which other people do not have. They are like professional healers in that they lay claim to special knowledge, but this knowledge is not always as formally recognized or organized as professional knowledge. Folk healers may work to professionalize their discipline – as has happened in some African countries with respect to African indigenous healing (Last & Chavunduka, 1989). It is, however, not always in the interests of folk healers to professionalize, especially as a common way of entering a folk-healing role is not through knowledge, which anyone can learn, but through an attribute which some people are seen to possess. A clairvoyant, for example, may need to have the 'gift of seeing' (being able to see the spiritual world), and a Zulu healer, expert in the treatment of *indiki* possession, may have experienced *indiki* possession herself (Ngubane, 1977).

When we look at what has been written about folk healing in the southern African context and, indeed, internationally, we enter into an area which is often misunderstood. We have seen from the previous chapter that there are a number of myths about mental illness in Africa – these extend into myths about indigenous healing. Most common among these is the view that all 'unsophisticated' Africans make use of the folk sector by choice, and that as they become more sophisticated, they turn to biomedicine (Swartz, 1986). Together with this view goes the belief that non-African people never use the folk sector, which is untrue. As is the case elsewhere in the world, there is increasing interest in the region in a wide range of folk therapies, including card reading, use of crystals, astrology, and so on. There is also considerable interest in African therapies, as can be seen by the popularity of books such as those by Bührmann (1984) and McCallum (1994).

Two major components of the folk sector in southern Africa are indigenous healing and healing through the African independent churches. There are many descriptions of indigenous and religious healing (Bührmann, 1981, 1983a; Bührmann & Gqomfa, 1981, 1982a, 1982b; Edwards, 1983a, 1983b; McCallum, 1994; Ngubane, 1977; Peltzer, 1995; Reynolds, 1996; West, 1975), and these will not be gone into in any detail here. Within African indigenous healing, a wide variety of healers exist, and they work in a range of contexts (Farrand, 1980; Mkhwanazi, 1986). Ngubane (1977), writing about healing in KwaZulu/Natal, distinguishes between an *inyanga* ('doctor') and an *isangoma* ('diviner'). The *inyanga* (generally a man) apprentices himself to another *inyanga* and through this learns to become a dispenser of herbal medicines. The *isangoma* is usually a woman who has been chosen by the ancestors to become a healer. On the path to becoming a healer, she will undergo a period of spirit possession, which is a necessary period of emotional disruption and will assist later with the development of clairvoyant powers. In addition to this spirit possession, there is apprenticeship training. Healing itself is undertaken using a variety of herbal remedies and rituals which may include music and dance as well as dream interpretation. Indigenous healing may take place on an outpatient or an inpatient basis, with the client living at the healer's home for a period (Peltzer, 1995).

Spirit possession as a path to becoming a healer has in the past been incorrectly identified as a form of psychopathology (Kruger, 1978), and many authors have stressed the culturally acceptable nature of a spirit possession illness in the process of a healer's development (Swartz, 1996). Although, as we have seen, there are many non-rational factors in the work of professional sector healers, biomedicine tends to emphasize rationality in its work and, in fact, to discount or refrain from reporting the non-rational aspects of healing – an approach which is in keeping with a very particular view of science (Gilbert & Mulkay, 1984; Turkle, 1995). The emphasis on non-rational aspects of healing in many aspects of folk sector practice, and in African indigenous healing in particular, can lead to the mistaken impression that there are no rules or rational procedures in such practices. Many studies show very clearly that rationality does play an important part in decision-making and treatment in African indigenous healing (Edwards, 1986; Reynolds, 1996).

Emphasis on the spiritual dimension is also central to healing in the African independent churches, which have a very large following in southern Africa (West, 1975). These churches often offer a synthesis between Christian beliefs and indigenous practices, though the churches differ on the degree to which they approve of belief in the power of the ancestors, and other factors central to African indigenous healing. Edwards (1983a, 1983b) provides detailed case material to show how healing in the Zionist church in the Eastern Cape province of South Africa incorporates both indigenous beliefs about posses-sion, and American Pentecostal church beliefs about similar issues, and about exorcism. Peltzer (1995: 191) indicates that in Zambia, Pentecostal churches offer an attractive healing environment for people dissatisfied with what they view as the one-sided care offered by biomedicine, and also with what they see as backward and commercially-oriented indigenous healing. Central to healing in these churches is the concept of being 'born again' as a Christian. Fundamentalist Christian churches, with an emphasis on healing through group ritual and prayer, have an enormous appeal across many social divides. The influence of television and North American 'televangelism' is also important.

An interesting feature of many folk-sector healing methods is that they occur publicly, and with a great deal of community participation. Some key cultural features of biomedicine – privacy and confidential-ity – are not necessarily as highly prized. The power of the group is used to understand and participate in the healing of problems. In the mental health field in particular, biomedicine's commitment to indi-vidual, private care breaks down to some degree. Group therapies, and even peer pressure, may be central to the professional treatment of addictions and personality problems. The central image of biomedi-cine, though, is that of the individual patient rather than the group.

Given the diversity and vibrancy of the folk sector, some central questions arise. First, how does the folk sector organize itself, and how does it relate to the professional sector? Second, what are different healing systems for? Third, how do people negotiate their way through the different sectors of care? We turn to these questions in the next two sections.

Intersectoral relationships and boundary issues

The professional sector, as we have seen, is well organized, and has ways of protecting its boundaries. In South Africa, for example, only psychologists registered with the Professional Board for Psychology (part of what used to be known as the South African Medical and Dental Council) may undertake certain psychological assessments. Only registered psychologists may call themselves psychologists. The same degree of legal protection is not offered to folk-sector practitioners – any person may claim to be an astrologer, for example, or an indigenous healer, without fear of legal reprisals.

Professions organize themselves partly to protect the public but also to protect themselves. Historically, the professions in southern Africa have been dominated by those with historical links with colonial powers, and it is hardly surprising that questions surrounding professionalization of indigenous healing have come to the fore in the postcolonial period (Last & Chavunduka, 1989). Over time, changes may occur as to whether a practice is regarded as professional or not. Thirty years ago, for example, anybody in South Africa who wished to do so could claim to be a clinical psychologist. Concerted and directed action by qualified psychologists helped to have the law changed. Other disciplines, such as homeopathy and chiropractic, have faced, and continue to face, different perceptions as to whether they are professions or not. As more therapies develop in the folk sector, should they become professional? Reflexology, iridology, and aromatherapy are examples of practices which have operated at the boundary in public consciousness between professional healing practices and lifestyle choices.

How do professional and folk healers interrelate? This is a crucial question for the public as people use both sectors. In general, mental health professionals are urged to respect folk-sector healing – African indigenous healing in particular (Swartz, 1996), and to recognize the contribution it makes to mental health care. Unfortunately, the political importance in post-apartheid South Africa of recognizing previously marginalized knowledge has also led to a lack of analysis of what different forms of indigenous healing can and cannot do (Swartz, 1996). Farmer (1997) has indicated that there are important public health implications of taking a romantic view of folk healing – it is necessary to be critical of all practices. He comments: 'If folk healing were so effective, the world's wealthy would be monopolizing it' (Farmer, 1997: 355). If a practice is culturally acceptable to a client, this does not necessarily mean that the practice is helpful to that client. The question of criteria for assessing a 'good' healing practice is discussed implicitly below.

What are healing systems for?

What are healing systems for? At face value, this seems a silly question with an obvious answer. Healing systems exist to make people better. But what do we mean when we talk of making people better? We have seen from the previous chapter that there are very different notions of normality and abnormality. There are also different cultural ideas about the relationship between the individual and society (Shweder & Bourne, 1982).

Even within professional healing, there may be very different ideas as to the aims of treatment. To put things crudely, a behaviourist psychologist may aim to change the client's behaviour, whereas an existential psychologist may wish to change the client's relationship with others in the world. In practice, both treatments may reach the same end, but there are differences in emphasis. Psychotherapy has developed within a culture of individualism, where individual personal growth and fulfilment are highly prized. Should we expect African indigenous healing, which has developed in a different context, to have the same aims?

All healing is only partly about the individual being healed. It is also about the maintenance and reproduction of the norms of a particular society. These norms may change dramatically over time, in accordance with broader cultural shifts. For example, until comparatively recently homosexuality was seen as a form of psychopathology within biomedicine, and it was considered appropriate to treat homosexuality as a mental disorder. We now regard homosexuality as a sexual variation rather than as a problem, and homosexuality itself is not a condition to be treated. Within some religious healing contexts, however, homosexuality is regarded as a sin or an affliction needing vigorous treatment. Depending on where a person is located with respect to different healing systems, and depending on the cultural beliefs of the person and those around him or her, a condition or life circumstance may or may not be seen as needing treatment.

Healing rituals may have such importance in terms of group needs that the question of whether an individual is being 'cured' by them may be secondary to the broader social function of healing. The contribution psychoanalysis has made to society is only partly the 'cures' of individuals (and, in fact, there are many questions about the efficacy of psychoanalysis relative to other treatments). What psychoanalysis has done, though, has been to provide a way of thinking about people and the world which has been highly influential – far beyond its influence in the consulting room.

Healing operates and is active in a political context as well. Comaroff (1985) has shown the role that healing practices have played in resistance under apartheid, and Lan (1984) and Reynolds (1996) have discussed the multiple roles of indigenous healers in the Zimbabwean liberation war. In South Africa, in the national reconstruction period, language heavily influenced by psychoanalysis is used to provide support for the Truth and Reconciliation Commission. As perpetrators and survivors of atrocities speak about what happened, though there is obviously concern that the process should be 'healing' for survivors, there is a more general concern that the Commission should provide a way in which an entire society can be healed (Owens, 1996), an issue which will be considered in more detail in Chapter 8. Gillian Slovo's (1997) account of her attempt to come to terms with her own history as the daughter of two of South Africa's most prominent political figures, one of whom was assassinated by the South African state, is clearly influenced by psychoanalytic ideas about the need for individuals to know about their past. But it is also part of the cultural landscape of a country trying to redefine itself.

It is a mistake, then, to think about healing systems only in terms of the immediate benefits they may or may not confer on individual clients. Healing systems also play a role in reinforcing and developing cultural norms and power bases, and in the political life of communities and nations. Just like education systems (which are there to educate) and legal systems (which are there to make and enact laws), they also have a function in the broader social and symbolic order. From this perspective, it is possible to view healing systems not only in terms of their ability to care, but also in terms of what they tell us about the society in which they operate. This does not, however, detract from their role for individuals who are suffering.

Paths to care

Let us return now to the question which opened this chapter: *What happens when somebody becomes mentally ill?* We can see now that the identification of a problem can lead to a wide range of behaviour on the part of the person(s) identified as having the problem, and on the part of those connected to the person(s) with the problem. Janzen (1978) described what he termed the 'quest for therapy' in what was then Zaïre, and he showed the large number of social factors involved in people's search for appropriate help.

Understanding how people move through different sites of care, and how they use different types of treatment simultaneously, is a challenge. We may have some difficulties in understanding the process if we assume that professional care is always better 'scientifically' than folk or popular sector care, and that folk healing is always 'culturally' more in tune with people than is professional care. In 1989, the following claim was made about black South Africans' use of healing systems:

> In general it is accepted that illnesses sent by the ancestors or the witches or caused by pollution cannot be treated within the Western system, and it is only when such treatments are unsuccessful that Western services are used. (My translation from Schoeman, 1989: 470; original in Afrikaans)

This quotation reveals some ambivalence regarding the folk sector, and regarding African people's use of it in particular. On the one hand, Schoeman claims Western therapies are unable to treat 'African illnesses'. On the other hand, when African therapies fail, then Western treatments are used. So professional healing is seen as both irrelevant to 'African' illnesses, and also a treatment of last resort. Part of the problem here is that Schoeman is, to an extent, stereotyping. Spiro (1991) has shown that many people who use biomedical mental health services, and not only those using them as a last resort, do not necessarily hold the same beliefs about illness and healing as those held by the practitioners. It is an oversimplification to expect that users of services will by choice use only those services which seem to share their world-view. First, people do not always have a choice – all too often, people have to use what is available, even if it is not exactly what they want or need. Second, there are many, and contradictory, world-views, not just one or two. So it is not possible to provide a 'Western' service for 'Western' people, and a 'non-Western' service for 'non-Western' people. The categories 'Western' and 'non-Western' are our creations, and reflect neither the diversity of beliefs (often mutually contradictory) that people hold, nor the commonalities that exist across apparently very different groups of people (Boonzaier & Sharp, 1988; Swartz, 1989). The plurality of resources used, furthermore, will also reflect the extent to which different systems of care can adequately address particular problems. Decision-making about which treatments to use is also not either rationally based or based on a detailed and explicated world-view. For example, at one time I was receiving three different treatments for a severe allergy: cortisone (from biomedicine), a treatment based on anthroposophical medicine (a form of healing with a spiritual component), and homeopathic remedies. I had faith in none of the three approaches to help me on its own, and I knew that practitioners from the three approaches would not approve of my using all three simultaneously but, probably quite irrationally, I thought that if I tried everything at once, it might work. (It did!) At that time, my discomfort was such that I was not thinking logically. I was also not acting in terms of any worked-out ideology of care. I was simply desperate. And this need for treatment, of some kind or another, together with what happens to be reasonably accessible to people, will help determine how people use resources.

Goldberg and Huxley (1980, 1992) have, for some time, been interested in the question of how people come to the attention of psychiatrists. They point out that it is not symptoms alone which determine the path to psychiatric care – a range of social factors can lead one person to a psychiatrist, and another, with the same symptom profile, never to see a psychiatrist. Focusing only on the professional sector in Britain, they show that factors which determine the path of people to the psychiatrist include the ways in which they themselves label their behaviour, the beliefs and abilities of general practitioners about mental disorders, and the availability of referral services. When services are scarce or inaccessible, for example, referral does not make much sense.

The Goldberg and Huxley (1992) model is relatively narrow in its focus and aimed specifically at understanding mental illness in the community in Britain. It is, however, possible to expand the model to include folk-sector healing (Gater et al., 1991). Parry & Swartz (1997: 239-241) have shown how the model can be used as a framework for exploring explanatory models and different beliefs about mental illness and how these impact upon people's decisions about use of mental health services. Ensink and Robertson (1996) have also explored the various types of healer used by people on their way to becoming psychiatric patients. One difficulty, though, in thinking about how people come to use psychiatric resources is that we may tend to think that formal psychiatric services are necessarily the end of the road in the quest for therapy for mental illness. What is probably more accurate is a picture of people using resources in a much less predictable way – moving back and forth amongst different types of healers (Spiro, 1991). The unpredictability does not imply randomness, or even, on all occasions, lack of rational judgement. Instead, it reflects people's search for help in a world not as rigidly organized as we professionals would like it to be. The search for treatment of and help with distress is not very different from the search for help with other issues affecting people's lives. Heap (1986) has shown how women in the informal settlement area of Khayelitsha near Cape Town make use in their daily lives of a variety of resources, both local and distant, depending on how easily and effectively networks can be accessed. Spiegel and Mehlwana (1997), furthermore, show how the concept of a household and of a supportive network changes and develops in the context of adversity and migration. Similarly, our choices about where to turn to for help with emotional distress will depend on what is available to us, and what seems to work.

In summary, we have seen in this chapter that mental illness and suffering is not just the domain of the professional sector. We have noted that different approaches to healing in this area have different emphases and ideologies, but that there are similarities and commonalities across approaches. People make use of resources according to what seems to be available and what seems to work. In the next section we shall turn to some particular conditions and issues in understanding mental health and illness in cultural perspective, before returning, at the end of the book, to broader issues affecting the way we work and the planning of policy.

PART III

Specific areas of interest

5

Depression and culture

Mr Carolus lives in a small rural community in South Africa. He is 32 years old, and for the past twelve years he has worked as a manual labourer for the same company. Three years ago, he was travelling in a bus which overturned. There were some serious injuries, but Mr Carolus was only slightly hurt. He was taken to a hospital along with other injured passengers. There he told the doctor on duty that his back was painful. The doctor did not feel it necessary to have Mr Carolus's back X-rayed, though he did arrange this for a number of the more seriously injured.

Mr Carolus describes this as a difficult time for him, especially as the accident happened shortly after his mother died. On returning to work, he found it difficult to continue with manual labour and was given less demanding physical work. This helped for some time, but soon he began to experience back pain. He consulted a doctor who examined him and could find nothing wrong. The pain persisted, and he returned to the doctor who again found nothing wrong. On his third visit the doctor became irritated and refused to examine Mr Carolus. He went to another primary health care facility, where there was a similar pattern of interaction. At various times, he was given mild analgesics for the pain, but it seemed clear that the primary health care personnel he saw did not feel there was very much wrong with his back. Sometimes, a doctor would book him off work for two days. This led to his being laughed at and teased by his superiors and colleagues as, according to them, real physical conditions were always given at least three days off – he must be faking.

I met Mr Carolus by chance as part of a survey we were doing – he had not been referred to me as a psychologist and had no idea what clinical psychologists do. He was a small, very thin, young-looking man with dark rings under his eyes. When I questioned him, he told me that he had lost a lot of weight and that he did not feel much like eating. He slept poorly, waking in the early hours and then was not able to go back to sleep. He cried quite regularly, and thought a lot about his dead mother. He was scared that he would lose his job and be unable to support his wife (who was pregnant). She was generally supportive but had also lost patience with him. His major concern, which he could not get out of his head, was that his injury from the bus accident was not being taken seriously. If only he had been X-rayed at the time, he could have received proper treatment and he would now be well. The thought of his not having been properly treated went round and round in his head and affected his concentration. He was also very tired all of the time.

I asked Mr Carolus about his mood. He said that he was not sad, and he seemed rather confused when I asked him if he thought he was depressed. He did not think so. He had on occasion thought that there might be something wrong with his nerves, but he knew that he was not crazy, and generally it was only women who suffered from their nerves. His only concern was his injury and the consequences of it. He spoke in a flat monotonous voice, and his face was typically that of a depressed person.

For ethical reasons, I could not simply collect the data from Mr Carolus and then leave. I therefore referred him back to the primary health care facility with a note to say that I thought Mr Carolus was suffering from depression and could probably benefit from a course of antidepressants. Some time later, I heard that he was feeling better and that his concerns about his back injury had abated, although they had not gone away completely.

How do we understand what has happened to Mr Carolus? Stories like his are not uncommon, and yet they challenge our ideas about mental health and illness, about the relationship between the mind and the body, and about what is appropriate health care. From a diagnostic point of view, we may think that Mr Carolus is depressed. The fact that he does not himself complain of a depressed mood does not exclude the diagnosis. The DSM-IV criteria for diagnosis of major depressive episode require five symptoms, one of which must be from the following group of symptoms, to a sufficient degree of severity:

- depressed mood
- appearing depressed / tearful to others
- loss of interest and pleasure in activities.

Mr Carolus seems sad and tearful (though he does not complain of being sad and depressed), he has lost weight, he has sleep problems, he seems to have concentration problems, he experiences fatigue. Paging through the DSM-IV we can consider other diagnoses – for example, those concerning anxiety. We could even explore posttraumatic stress disorder, given the accident Mr Carolus has survived.

What do we make of the pain, and the physical component to Mr Carolus's experiences? Once again, we can navigate the DSM-IV and look for disorders which include concern with the body and with bodily ailments. The introduction to the DSM-IV section on somatoform disorders contains the following, which seems to fit Mr Carolus rather well:

> The common feature of the Somatoform Disorders is the presence of physical symptoms that suggest a general medical condition (hence the term **somatoform**) and are not fully explained by a general medical condition, by the direct effects of a substance, or by another mental disorder ... The symptoms must cause clinically significant distress or impairment in the social, occupational, or other areas of functioning ... [T]he physical symptoms are not intentional (i.e. under voluntary control) ... [T]here is no diagnosable medical condition to fully account for the physical symptoms ... These disorders are often encountered in general medical settings. (DSM-IV, 1994: 445)

On the other hand, we are told in the DSM-IV information on mood episodes that 'in some cultures, depression may be experienced largely in somatic terms, rather than with sadness or guilt' (DSM-IV, 1994: 324). So perhaps Mr Carolus is depressed after all, with what the DSM-IV (1994: 324) would term *specific culture features*.

We could go on trying to argue the merits of various diagnoses for Mr Carolus, but this would probably not affect the treatment he would receive in the context of rural primary health care in South Africa. Even when highly sophisticated psychiatric services are available, the diagnosis itself would probably not dramatically alter the approach to treatment.

So far we have only looked at the diagnostic possibilities. What about the treatment Mr Carolus has received? Do we know for certain he has been adequately helped from a medical point of view? Would an X-ray at the time of the accident indeed have shown some treatable physical damage? Has there begun to be a pattern whereby Mr Carolus is seen as a 'difficult' patient and whereby he does not receive the full and serious attention of health care personnel? This is a common complaint on the part of people experiencing chronic pain (Good et al., 1992). Perhaps he is operating at the boundaries of what medicine can do for people – many very caring physicians recognize that chronic pain may be extremely difficult to treat, however seriously the symptoms are taken. Kleinman (1995b:133) speaks of 'demoralization as an intersubjective process of suffering shared by patient, family and practitioners' in which all can feel helpless in the face of chronic pain.

There is also a question about the link between the diagnostic possibilities and the health care Mr Carolus has received. For example, the DSM-IV speaks about there being no *diagnosable* medical condition. There is a difference, surely, between there being a diagnosable condition (theoretically, and in the best of all possible worlds) and one that has been diagnosed, in the real world of care available to Mr Carolus. Possibly, the diagnosis could change if the health care available to Mr Carolus changed. The authors of the DSM-IV would no doubt argue (correctly) that they can base categories only on the assumption of adequate medical care available, but the DSM-IV is often used where resources are so limited that this condition is not met. Technically, this may invalidate the use of the DSM-IV, but practically, the primary care personnel faced with Mr Carolus and his life situation have to provide the care that they can – and diagnose as best they can. But there is another complication. According to the DSM-IV (1994: 445), as we have seen above, 'These disorders are often encountered in general medical settings'. It is our task, as students of culture and mental health, to explore how this happens. It is not enough to say that the disorders 'are encountered' – we need to ask who encounters them, and why. We need to understand why people who come to general medical settings sometimes present themselves in this way, and to understand what the symptoms tell us not only about the people who present them, but also about the relationships between these people and the systems they go to for help.

Mr Carolus's illness experience poses challenges for us in the ways in which it asks questions about the disease categories we use, and the assumptions we make about how the world is ordered. In this and the following chapter, we shall look at two related issues – how we understand depression cross-culturally, and how we think about the use of the body as a way of experiencing and expressing distress. Concerns with depression and with somatic expressions of distress have been central in debates on culture and mental health, and it is useful to discuss aspects of these now, as they will be relevant in discussions of other areas as well.

Thinking about depression and the emotions cross-culturally

The term 'depression' can be used in many ways. It can refer to a *mood* – the feeling of being depressed. It can refer to a *symptom* of a range of psychiatric and other disorders – for example, a substantial proportion of people suffering from schizophrenia experience feelings of depression at some stage of the illness (Elk et al., 1986; Jones et al., 1994). It can also refer to a *psychiatric disease* or *mental disorder* in its own right (Kleinman & Good, 1985b: 2). Kleinman and Good (1985b) point out how the confusion between these different uses of the term may create confusion for cross-cultural researchers. We have seen, for example, that according to the DSM-IV, the subjective experience of depressed mood is not a necessary criterion for the diagnosis of a major depressive episode. So one person, when talking about depression cross-culturally, may be talking about an experience of a mood or symptom, and another may be talking about a mental disorder in which the subjective experience of that depressed mood or symptom is not necessarily present. Some of the implications of this difference will become clear later in this section.

The experience of feeling sad and depressed is very common (Robins & Reiger, 1992), and generally quite easy to recognize within one's own social group. For this reason, as Littlewood and Lipsedge (1997: 61) point out, 'precisely because sadness or happiness are everyday occurrences, we already have available cultural mechanisms for understanding them, for modifying them and for incorporating them into our social life'. By extension, we also may have difficulty in understanding how these feelings, which are so much part of our own cultural experience, are experienced by others. We may also have difficulty accepting that it is possible for people with different emotional styles to experience these feelings at all. I was once involved in a group situation in which two of the participants were both white South African women in their sixties. One of the women was part of a religious community which was known to encourage free expression of the emotions; the other belonged to a group in which the norm was more reserved. When the sister of the second woman died suddenly, the first woman said that people from the more reserved religious group did not experience emotions fully, and that we should not be overly concerned – death was not a big issue for them. Understandably, the woman who had lost her sister suddenly, and was all but frozen with grief, felt angry and misunderstood. There are many possible reasons for her callous treatment by the woman from the expressive religious group, and the remark was definitely unfair and unkind. Part of what made the remark possible, though, was an interpretation of different subcultural styles of expressing and dealing with emotions.

As we will see below, there are a number of ways of looking at depression cross-culturally. We will consider first an *evolutionist* approach, followed by a *meaning-centred* approach. This leads to a discussion of changing beliefs about the extent of depression in Africa. Finally, we will think about the apparent tensions between seeing depression as a biological condition as opposed to a social one.

The evolutionist approach

In situations of oppression, racism, or war, there is much to be gained, and very little to be lost, by either side minimizing the emotional experience of the other. As we have seen in Chapter 4, the development of psychiatry in southern Africa was very much bound up with the history of colonization, with the early psychiatrists coming from the colonizing powers. The following quotation gives some idea of how psychiatry, as practised by whites in the USA, was elaborated in the context of racial oppression in that country:

> Naturally, most of the [negro] race are care-free, live in the 'here and now' with a limited capacity to recall or profit by experiences of the past. Sadness and depression have little part in his psychological make-up. (Bevis, 1921; as quoted by Littlewood & Lipsedge, 1997: 61)

Here, psychiatric knowledge can serve to legitimate cruel practices – if sadness and depression have little part in black people's psychological make-up, then there is less worry about hurting them emotionally. It also, coincidentally, can be used to block the advancement of black people in the world of work – people who are 'care-free' and live only in the present are not the sort of people who should be given too much responsibility. There has even been South African psychological research on 'the work-shy coloured man', research which could in a macabre way be seen to apply to people like Mr Carolus (Potgieter, 1986). We can see here the clear link between economic oppression and the viewing of black people as psychologically 'other' – in fact, as psychologically less sophisticated than whites.

It is difficult to translate the term 'depression' into all languages in the world, because of different idioms of distress in different cultures. Drennan et al. (1991) report that in their attempt to translate a well-known assessment tool into Xhosa, they had difficulties with translation of the word 'sad'. A Xhosa-speaking psychologist translated the word 'sad' as *khatazekile*. On back-translation by two senior students of African languages, *khatazekile* was translated as 'worried'. Sadness and worry have, from a psychiatric point of view, very different implications for diagnosis and treatment, as sadness may be a key symptom in depression, with worry a feature of an anxiety state. This difficulty in translating sadness has been experienced in many contexts (Kleinman & Good, 1985a). An important question is how different researchers make sense of the difficulties. One of the more controversial writers on the topic is Leff (1981, 1988), whose earlier formulations met with extensive criticism (Kleinman & Good, 1985b).

Leff (1988) reports that in Britain, patients are less likely to differentiate depression from anxiety than are psychiatrists. He reports on a study which shows that psychiatrists expected that patients would distinguish far more clearly between depression and anxiety than patients in fact did (Leff, 1988: 71). Psychiatrists anticipated that patients would say there is no overlap at all between feelings of depression and those of anxiety, whereas patients experienced quite a considerable overlap between the two emotions. As Leff points out, psychiatrists are harbouring 'idealised disease concepts, despite the fact that patients usually exhibit a mixture of the symptoms considered characteristic of each type of neurosis' (Leff, 1988: 71). Leff's conclusion to this and similar findings is instructive:

> ... English patients still have a considerable way to go in achieving a clear distinction between anxiety, depression and anger. On the other hand, psychiatrists have crystallised quite different conceptions of these unpleasant emotions. It is not surprising to find that they are at the leading edge of this process of emotional differentiation, where they act not only as pioneers, but also as educators. (Leff, 1988: 72)

It is interesting to note that Leff's conclusion here is not that psychiatrists are wrong – that they do not fully understand that their categories of emotion do not fit as well as they could with those of their patients. Instead, Leff here has a hierarchy of understanding the emotions, and at the top of the hierarchy – at the 'leading edge' as Leff puts it – are psychiatrists. From one important perspective, this is a good thing. If psychiatrists are those who are entrusted professionally with making sure that people's mental health is at its best, then surely they should know more than the average person about the emotions. In another way, though, Leff's argument is worrying. There is no evidence at all that experiencing anxiety and depression as separate illness categories is of any benefit to people. Why should the 'process of emotional differentiation', as Leff calls it, be a good thing? Clearly, Leff is setting great store by some of the cultural values which underlie Western society, and those which underlie biomedicine in particular. In the post-Freudian Western world, having a language which differentiates between different emotions is highly prized. Within Western culture, furthermore, great store has been set, for a long time, by the understanding of things by breaking them into smaller and smaller parts, and the model of the machine made up of smaller and smaller components has been used to develop understandings not only of mechanical things, but also of people. That there are problems with this way of seeing the world has become increasingly clear in the human sciences, and also within a world increasingly reliant on computer simulation for the development of knowledge (Turkle, 1995; Young, 1980). But much of Western thinking, and the success of Western technology, has depended on this way of seeing the world. Within biomedicine, the idea that the body functions like a machine, different parts of which can be analysed separately, has also been spectacularly successful (Gordon, 1988). Hence, as we have seen in Chapter 3, psychiatry's concern with fine-grained diagnostic decision-making, and Leff's belief that being able to differentiate between emotions is of value.

Professional mental health practices operate best with a high degree of diagnostic specificity and with differentiation of emotional states, partly because of their construction within the cultural norms described above. But Leff's argument, which places psychiatry at the developmental high point of English cultural understanding of emotions, confuses disease and illness. Within psychiatry, the more differentiated the emotions are, the better, as diagnosis and treatment (to an extent) depend on this differentiation. But there is no reason to assume that experiencing one's emotions in a form which is familiar to psychiatrists is any better or more sophisticated than any other way. The only way in which it is helpful to feel the way a psychiatrist might expect one to feel (and this is not unimportant) is that this may make it easier to access whatever help the psychiatrist may be able to give. But good transcultural psychiatry should, as Murphy (1977) said, 'begin at home'. In other words, if we are to understand mental health practices in cultural context, we need to see how those practices are culturally informed, and not to assume that they are the best way of seeing the world, even in 'Western' culture.

The value Leff places on the differentiation of the emotions in the style of Western psychiatry puts the Western psychiatrist at the end point of a developmental or evolutionary process whereby people come to experience their emotions in more and more psychiatric terms. But what about people whose experiences are very different? It is not surprising that in earlier work Leff (1981) saw the development of emotional differentiation as parallel to a process whereby people moved from 'traditional' to 'modern' ways of being, and from a more group-oriented to a more individualistic culture. Once again, the 'modern' way of doing things is seen as further along a developmental scale than is the 'traditional' way. Part of the problem with this evolutionist (Shweder & Bourne, 1982) view of understanding how people and societies develop is that it once again specifies an end point for emotional development. 'Traditional' people are seen to use the body more for emotional expression, and it is assumed that as they become more sophisticated they will experience the world more in psychological ways. We shall return to this issue from another perspective in Chapter 10.

In the light of some criticisms of his work (Kleinman & Good, 1985b), Leff (1988) revised some of his earlier views about the development of emotional differentiation, and there can be no doubt as to his seriousness about and contribution to our understanding of mental health practices internationally. What is instructive, though, in reading his carefully-argued accounts of the emotions, is the echo of very simplistic statements like that of Bevis (1921) quoted earlier. Bevis (1921) talks of the 'limited capacity' of the 'negro', and his typically not feeling 'sadness'. Just as Leff places the psychiatrist in the position of 'educator' and 'pioneer', so Bevis places the white American higher along the path of emotional and moral development than the 'negro'. We could, in fact, infer from the literature a hierarchy of sophistication which would look something like that shown in Figure 5.1:

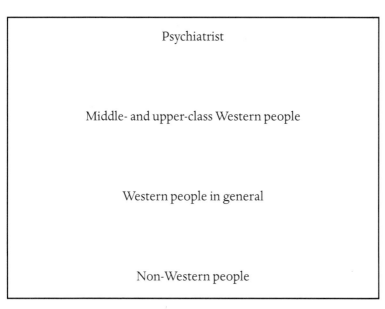

Psychiatrist

Middle- and upper-class Western people

Western people in general

Non-Western people

Figure 5.1 A hierarchy of understanding of the emotions implied in some accounts of cross-cultural psychiatry

Generally speaking, those who hold with this implicit view do not have any desire other than to help as many people as possible – it is easy to think of this way of seeing things as evidence of crude racism, which is not always fair. But the consequences of this evolutionist view may be serious. I have shown elsewhere (Swartz, 1985b,1986, 1987b) how it was possible for the emotional experiences of migrant mineworkers in South Africa to be interpreted in terms of their difficulties in adapting to a 'modern' or 'Westernized' lifestyle. This formulation, which fits in well with the stereotypes of Figure 5.1, ignored or glossed over the inhumane conditions under which migrant workers lived. These conditions alone, and not any problems in dealing with the demands of the 'modern', 'Western' world, could account for many difficulties in adjustment.

There are two ways, then, in which the evolutionist model of the emotions works. First, emotions such as depression are seen to be the realm of sophisticated people, as unsophisticated people cannot experience such feelings. Second, when 'unsophisticated' people do come to experience psychological symptoms, this is as a result of an unnatural or premature contact with, or immersion in, the modern or sophisticated world. Modernity (or Westernization), which brings with it all the material benefits of the modern world, is also seen as psychologically dangerous for those at the edges of society. Neither of these ways of seeing the emotions gives sufficient credence to the complex emotional states which are experienced outside of dominant Western culture.

A meaning-centred approach

The first step in creating a culturally informed view of depression and the emotions is a recognition of the diversity of emotional experience in different contexts. For very many people, for example, the experience of depression is a negative thing, and to be avoided or treated if at all possible. Obeyesekere (1985), however, shows that within a Buddhist society, the very feelings of hopelessness we associate with a pathological condition – depression – are desired feeling states. Buddhists, Obeyesekere (1985: 134) argues, *aim* to find the hopelessness in their world, and in the world as a whole. It is only through recognition of this hopelessness that salvation becomes possible. In Obeyesekere's (1985) rendering of Buddhist ideology, therefore, depression can become an ideologically acceptable mode of being and a path to true understanding.

What is striking about Obeyesekere's analysis is that he is speaking of a non-Western cultural experience of what we would call depression, which does not conform with the preferred Western norm. It is also very difficult to dismiss this emotional experience as either 'primitive' or 'undifferentiated'. There are many other examples of ways in which the emotions are experienced in different countries, which reinforce this view. In discussing the experience of emotion in Iran, Good (1977) discusses what he terms 'the semantics of illness' – a network of meaning around suffering and illness which, in Iran, is associated with feelings of the heart. The overriding importance of this meaning-centred approach is less in the specifics it tells us about depression and the emotions in any specific country, than about an approach to elaborating the meaning of emotions in any context. Lutz (1985) points out that differentiations of emotions in different cultures take on many forms. It is very difficult for outsiders to differentiate the emotion *fago* ('compassion/love/sadness') from *lalomweiu* ('loneliness/sadness'), but the distinction is meaningful to the Ifaluk of Micronesia, amongst whom such emotional experiences occur. This difficulty (which even a Western psychiatrist would face) does not make the outsider unsophisticated about emotions in general – just uninformed about emotions in Micronesia. Similarly, vast numbers of people are uninformed about how Western psychiatry thinks about emotions.

When we are told, then, for example, that guilt may be less of a feature of depression in non-Western cultures than in the West, or that sadness may be replaced by bodily complaints, our task is not to look for the ways in which some people may not fulfil standard biomedical criteria of what constitutes depression. It is rather to attempt to understand what the particular pattern of symptoms means in the context within which the person lives. Interestingly, this way of looking at things helps us solve the difficult problem of how to think about someone who suffers from what we would call a depressive illness but who does not experience depressed mood. Our categories (such as those given by the DSM-IV) are useful in that they form the basis of biomedical interventions, but they are clearly not sufficient in a culturally informed analysis, nor should they be at the centre of one. When we consider people who are depressed (in our terms) without feeling sad or guilty, and who may experience various pains and symptoms in their bodies, we open the way to thinking of suffering and unhappiness as it plays itself out in people's lives, lives which are not bound by our categories. As we feel more comfortable with relegating our (very useful) labels and interpretations to their rightful place, not at centre stage, we can begin to think about suffering and pain – emotional and physical – more empathically and creatively (Kleinman, 1986, 1995b).

How does this type of analysis help us understand Mr Carolus, whose story opened this chapter? First, and very importantly, we need to recognize that though finding a diagnosis for Mr Carolus may be useful to us, it does not tell us the whole story. His experiences are elaborated in a context which, if we want to understand him fully, we shall also have to try to understand. What is it like to be a manual labourer living in the small town he lives in? What did his mother mean to him? What is the meaning of work in this community? How is the health system, and interaction with it, viewed by people in the community? It may not be possible, given time and other resource constraints, to find out much in response to these questions, but the important thing about having these questions in our heads is that we do not reduce Mr Carolus to someone who fits more or less well into our categories of depression. We shall look later at how people like Mr Carolus challenge our categories which distinguish body from mind.

Changing views on the extent of depression in Africa

There has, over the past thirty years, been a dramatic difference in professionals' views on the extent of depression in Africa. Previously, it was thought to be rare. Nowadays, it is thought, if anything, to be more common even than in Europe and North America. Part of the reason for this change is simple – there have been many more epidemiological studies which have shown this pattern over recent years (Abas & Broadhead, 1997; Parry, 1996). Littlewood and Lipsedge (1997: 67-68) suggest three possibilities as to why depression used to be seen as rare amongst non-Europeans:

1 Depressive illnesses did occur but they were not noticed.
2 Depression was missed because it didn't appear to the Europeans as depression.

3 There has been a real change and depression is now more common.

I shall briefly consider each of these possibilities in turn.

1   Why depression may have been overlooked

Littlewood and Lipsedge (1997: 68) argue that in the context of few psychiatric facilities, only people with socially disruptive behaviour are likely to come to the attention of mental health services. People who are violent or get into trouble with the law will almost always get noticed, but people who are depressed and essentially bother nobody but themselves tend to be overlooked. Littlewood and Lipsedge argue further that where there have been very poor services in the colonial context, depressed people may have been reluctant to go for help.

My own clinical work and research in psychiatric hospitals catering for black South Africans (Swartz, 1991a) corroborates this view. Almost all patients who came to be admitted to psychiatric care were causing problems for people around them, or were engaged in socially inappropriate behaviour, such as walking about naked. A person who was simply depressed and unhappy was almost never seen. At that time, community psychiatric services for black South Africans hardly existed to any meaningful extent, so there was effectively nowhere within the professional mental health system for depressed people to go. Let us think back to the operation of the Goldberg and Huxley (1992) model of paths to psychiatric inpatient care discussed in Chapter 4. Perhaps, in South Africa, depression was not picked up at primary health care level. Many studies have shown that primary health care practitioners may not be very good at detecting psychiatric morbidity, of which, at the primary health care level, depression is a major part (Parry & Swartz, 1997; Reeler, 1987). This may not always be because such practitioners lack the ability to detect disorder, though this is certainly a factor. In conducting interviews preparatory to studies on psychological factors in primary health care in a South African village (Miller & Swartz, 1990a; Reynolds & Swartz, 1993), I found that even practitioners who could detect depression and similar problems were reluctant to do so. One doctor who spoke to me described his difficulty as 'It's just me and my pills here'. He knew that the emotional problems he was seeing needed the help of someone who had the time and skills of a person like a mental health practitioner, such as a social worker or a psychiatric professional nurse, but there were none who had more than a few hours a month to spare (at best) for an entire community. In this context, he felt, it was better for him not to begin to open up painful areas for discussion with patients as all that would happen would be that they would become upset, with no possibility of further help from professionals. Here, then, is an example of non-detection of depression for one of the reasons Littlewood and Lipsedge (1997) suggest.

A corollary to the Littlewood and Lipsedge (1997) argument is that one can expect there to be more cases of depression emerging as services become more accessible and appropriate – and this is what has been hoped will indeed happen in a postcolonial situation. (Unfortunately, resource constraints and a lack of prioritizing of mental health issues throughout the world may have often made this hope rather hollow – see Desjarlais et al., 1995.) Epidemiological community-based studies may help detect cases which would otherwise be hidden. These studies do not depend on depressed people coming for help or being seen as depressed by unqualified or under-resourced primary health care personnel. Gillis (1992) found the rate of depression amongst elderly women in an informal settlement near Cape Town was as high as 40 per cent – in an area in which, at the time, there was very little in the way of mental health care. Shortly after this, Binedell (1993) conducted a study amongst community health workers, some of them working in the same area where Gillis (1992) had conducted the survey. These community health workers were all being employed by community-based health organizations committed to optimal health services for all South Africans. These organizations and community health workers were working in the context of progressive attempts to begin to build appropriate health services for those who had been denied them through the apartheid health system. Interestingly, the community health workers, practically without exception, told Binedell that depression was not a problem in their areas. They said this even if they worked where the Gillis (1992) study had taken place. Binedell was careful to use a methodology based on case stories, so that the non-detection of depression was not owing to the community health workers' unfamiliarity with psychiatric terms. According to the community health workers, mental disorders which were seen in their areas were confined only to socially disruptive conditions of the type I have mentioned above. Clearly, if detection is to become adequate within a revamped health care system, the issue of training for primary health care personnel will have to be carefully thought about. This is something we shall return to towards the end of this book.

2 Depression taking on different forms

Littlewood and Lipsedge (1997: 69) point out that guilt seems to be a less common feature of depression in West Africa than it is in Britain, and that hallucinations may be a feature of West African depression. As we have seen, the DSM-IV also mentions absence of guilt as characteristic of depression in come cultures. Hallucinations (sensory experiences of phenomena which are not objectively present) are characteristic of psychosis in Britain, but may appear even in mild depression in West Africa. The second major feature Littlewood and Lipsedge (1997: 69) identify as important in looking at different forms of depression is the use of the body for the expression of emotional distress – this issue, which has been raised earlier, will be considered in more detail later in the chapter.

Recently, Rumble and her colleagues (1996) conducted South Africa's first ever two-stage survey of mental illness in a community. The standard research instrument used was the ninth edition of the *Present State Examination* (PSE) (Wing et al., 1974), which has been extensively used internationally, including for the *International Pilot Study of Schizophrenia* (WHO, 1973). When results were first analysed, it appeared that there was an exceptionally high rate of psychosis in the community. When the researchers looked more closely at their data, however, they found that a number of respondents who were depressed had attributed their depression to the wrongdoing of others, including witchcraft. When this was rated in the PSE scoring system, it was seen as evidence of paranoid symptoms of psychosis. On further examination, though, it appeared that blaming others for misfortune, including believing that one may be bewitched, is a culturally acceptable model for explaining misfortune in that community. When Rumble et al. (1996) re-analysed their data, they found that the rate of psychosis dropped and the rate of depression rose. There are at least two ways to interpret what has happened here, from a research point of view. Rumble et al. (1996) contend that features of the *Present State Examination* scoring system would tend to encourage over-diagnosis of psychosis (and hence under-diagnosis of milder depressions and anxiety states) in contexts such as South Africa (cf. Swartz et al., 1985). Another interpretation is that Rumble et al. (1996) should have known before they conducted their study what the cultural norms were in their community and therefore should not have rated as psychiatric *symptoms* people's culturally acceptable (but 'paranoid' to an outsider) explanations of their misfortune. By definition, a symptom which reaches the proportion of delusion must be out of keeping with the norms of the person's culture. Either way, the Rumble et al. (1996) study reminds us, as do a number of others from Africa (Binitie, 1971; Sijuwola, 1995), that apparently paranoid features may mask features of depression.

This type of observation may indeed explain why depression may have been missed in Africa in the past, and it may also account for why depression, as we have seen, has been thought to be rare amongst African psychiatric patients in South Africa (Freed & Bishop, 1980; Gijana & Louw, 1981; Luiz, 1981). In at least some of these cases, depression could have been misdiagnosed on the basis of apparently psychotic features such as hallucinations and delusions – precisely those features which are most likely to catch the attention of mental health services, especially when services are insufficient to meet all the professional mental health needs of a country. Even when there is no doubt about the primary diagnosis of a psychotic disorder, clinicians may not enquire fully enough about the presence of treatable depressive symptoms as part of what is bothering the patient (Elk et al., 1986).

3   Patterns of depression may be changing

Patterns of mental illness change over time. Leff (1988: 60-61), for example, shows how hysteria has, over a period of thirty years, accounted for a smaller and smaller percentage of admissions to psychiatric hospitals in Britain. Similarly, there may have been a genuine increase in depression in Africa over decades. Depression is quite common in later life, as Littlewood and Lipsedge (1997: 68) point out, and this is borne out by local studies (Ben-Arie et al., 1987; Gillis, 1992). As the life expectancy in Africa increases, we can expect to see more and more depression.

If the information were available, we could quite easily test this theory by examining the relationship between rates of depression and age. If we could find, for example, that there were indeed more cases of depression over time, and that these cases were amongst old people, of whom there are more than there were previously, then we could attribute the changes to a longer-surviving population. We could conduct further studies in which we could examine depression in different age bands. This would help us find out whether only greater life expectancy gave rise to higher numbers of depressed people, or whether there were changes in the number of cases amongst younger people as well.

Unfortunately, accurate epidemiological data not available to enable us to undertake such studies; even well-designed comprehensive studies are difficult to undertake at present as they are very expensive. So we are left with the greater life-expectancy hypothesis as one which cannot be fully investigated retrospectively. It is difficult to know for sure whether patterns of depression are in fact changing, and what such changes might mean. If we begin, as far as we are able, to collect valid data now, we can begin to track changes into the future. The past, as far as the history of depression in Africa is concerned, is difficult to interpret from our current perspective.

This discussion of changes in rates of depression, though, may tend to reify (see Chapter 1) depression into an entity or a 'thing' which can be 'discovered' in the world out there, and it is important to consider ways in which the influence of this reification may affect how we think about depression in cultural context. In this regard, it is useful to look at some of the thinking that exists around depression as a biological entity.

Depression: biological or social and cultural?

The enormous strides made in genetics and in biological psychiatry hold out hope for millions of patients around the world, and with good reason. With new research methods, and with the technology available, diagnostic accuracy has improved and new-generation treatments – such as powerful antidepressants – are available. One of these antidepressants, Prozac, has changed perceptions, in the USA in particular, as to what psychopharmacology can achieve. The Prozac phenomenon has become part of a realignment in the way that suffering is viewed in that country (Kramer, 1993; Wurtzel, 1994). Viewing these developments from the perspective of those working in low-income countries, it is possible to be both unrealistically gloomy and unrealistically hopeful about what this means for us. An unrealistically gloomy view is that mainstream psychiatry in Europe and North America is becoming so dependent on expensive technology and biological treatments that there will be little benefit to low-income countries. An unrealistically hopeful view is that psychiatry will develop cheap and effective drugs which will be easily applicable internationally and will, in all probability, make our concerns about culture and mental health irrelevant.

Tensions between biological and sociocultural understandings of psychopathology occur throughout studies of mental disorders. Discussions about depression, however, have been at the centre of this debate. This is partly because of the great successes there have been in the biological understanding and treatment of mood disorders – depression, and its partner, mania, a condition characterized by inappropriately elated mood. Another reason for the interest in depression in this context is that it represents a mood state with which very many people can identify. A third reason is that depression, as we have seen, can be difficult to detect, especially in a diverse society. It is quite easy to see when someone's behaviour is socially disruptive, but depression is often not obvious. Depression is also commonly associated with suicide (though, in fact, a proportion of people with other mental disorders kill themselves; Jones et al., 1994), and the hope exists that if there could be some easy way of diagnosing and treating depression biologically, the tragedy of suicide could be prevented.

There may be unfortunate consequences of expecting the successes of biological psychiatry to do too much for us, as the following example shows. Some years ago I was working as part of a psychiatric research group focusing on cultural and social issues in many disorders, including depression. A substantial proportion of the people being studied were Xhosa-speaking, and there was little expertise in Xhosa in the research group. We have already seen in this chapter and in Chapter 2 how difficult it can be to diagnose depression accurately through an interpreter, especially where the client speaks a language very different from one's own. At the time, the dexamethasone suppression test (DST) was being welcomed by some as a valid diagnostic tool for major depression. This is a blood test, and the evidence for its ability to identify depression from a range of other conditions, or to differentiate between different forms of depression, is still being debated (Blouin et al., 1992; Howland & Thase, 1991; Koyama & Yamashita, 1992; Parker et al., 1995; Ribeiro et al., 1993). What is important for the current discussion is not the diagnostic strengths and weaknesses of the DST, but how it was seen by some. One of my colleagues suggested that our diagnostic difficulties were over. We could simply use the DST to assess depression, we could then treat with antidepressants, and our problems would be solved.

Assessing depression only in this way would enable researchers and clinicians to get directly to the disease of depression, as carefully defined, using a biological diagnostic instrument. They would be looking for the mental disorder of depression regardless of whether the person subjectively felt depressed or not. This way of thinking is an example of trying to develop a way of dealing with patients without having to talk to them – an ideal which offers clinicians the (false) hope of a precise science (cf. Sullivan, 1986). Put in another way, it is an attempt to get at the disease of depression without giving any regard to the illness experience. Kleinman (1988) speaks of the tendency within psychiatric thinking to believe that the biology of depression and anxiety disorders underwrites the inner form of these disorders, but cultural beliefs and values so shape the 'expression' of the disease that the bodily complaints come to 'mask' the 'real' psychiatric disease 'underlying' them. Indeed, at one point the term 'masked depression' was widely used to indicate this phenomenon. (Kleinman, 1988: 25)

The belief that only the disease is real, and the illness just an illusion, is attractive within biomedical thinking but, as we have seen in Chapter 1, is not tenable. What then do we make of the biological evidence in depression? Clearly, the answer is that we should not have to choose between the patient's disease and the illness. Both are realities, and both require attention. As Kleinman and Good (1985b) point out, depression is both biological and social, and it is a mistake to believe that if one takes the biological approach seriously that one must ignore the illness experience. The DST cannot tell us about the illness experience of depression, nor was it designed to do so. A moving testimony to the importance of understanding the feelings and the experience of living with depression and other forms of suffering can be found in a book by Jamison (1995). Jamison is a recognized authority in the field of mood disorders, and believes that biological understanding is very important and necessary. As a sufferer from a mood disorder herself, though, she is able to give important insights into the necessity for there being a caring and meaning-centred dimension to how people with such disorders should be treated.

The promise of biological understanding, then, to strip away the issues we have to face in understanding depression cross-culturally, is an illusion. The challenge to understand what is happening with people's bodies and emotions to express their feelings and their life circumstances becomes stronger, and not weaker, the more we know about the biology of depression (cf. Eisenberg, 1986; 1995). It is interesting, though, that some of the heated debate about the use of the DST diagnostically has been in the assessment of depression amongst mentally handicapped people (Mattes & Amsell, 1993; Mudford et al., 1995; Soni et al., 1992). Some mentally handicapped people have severe difficulties communicating, and one can understand why some practitioners have wanted to find a way of assessing depression without having to communicate with the handicapped people. There is a parallel between this wish and the wish on the part of my colleague to diagnose depression in Xhosa-speaking people without having to deal with all the language difficulties involved. We have seen earlier in this chapter how it was once thought that 'unsophisticated' people could not feel depression. The 'masked depression' hypothesis has shifted this to the view that 'unsophisticated' people may indeed feel depression, but they may not know it – hence the use of the body for expression of emotion. A less damning version of this view may be that some people experience depression but we as clinicians do not know an easy way to find this out. A similar argument can be made regarding the problems in assessing depression amongst severely and profoundly mentally handicapped people. We can see, then, that there could be similarities between the way mental health workers view cultural and linguistic difference and the way they view mental handicap. If difference is not carefully thought about, it can easily come to be seen as deficit. Interestingly, Sinason (1992) has shown how mentally handicapped people can come to develop what she terms 'secondary handicap' in response to the way they are treated. Treatment which can contribute to this 'secondary handicap' – the mentally handicapped persons' not making the best use of the resources and intelligence they do have – includes well-meaning but patronizing care. Sinason (1992) is able to show, through her careful meaning-centred work with mentally handicapped people, that they are able to experience and to communicate a far wider range of emotions – including depression – than many thought possible. The challenge, then, in looking at depression in diverse groups will always include the challenge to understand what life with depression is like.

We have seen in this section and earlier chapters that the idea that suffering can be reduced to a bodily experience alone is central to some ways of thinking within mental health care and within biomedicine in general. We also know that the intellectual tradition of focusing on the body as a machine separate from the mind, which goes back centuries (Gordon, 1988), has led to some of biomedicine's greatest achievements. Partly because of these achievements, and because of the difficulties we face understanding the emotions cross-culturally, it may be tempting to see depression and the emotions in purely physical terms. This would lead us to ignoring the illness experience so important to a full understanding. There is a tendency to believe that the exciting strides being made in biological psychiatry mean that the social and cultural dimensions of illness are relatively unimportant (Eisenberg, 1995). There is some irony in the fact that there seem to be two very different trends of thought amongst mental health practitioners regarding the body as a site for the experience and expression of the emotions. On the one hand, there is an increasing tendency towards naïve biologism in some areas of psychiatric thought (Eisenberg, 1995). On the other hand, mental health practitioners continue to see people who experience suffering and distress through the body as, by definition, unsophisticated, and certainly less sophisticated than those who experience distress in more psychological terms. The language of the body, so valued by mental health workers in one sense, is devalued by them in another. This irony can be seen to be at the centre of many debates in the field of culture and mental health, and will be considered further when we look at somatization in the next chapter.

6
Speaking with the body: somatization

Mr Jaxa is a 20-year-old man who has recently moved from a rural area to a large South African city. Unable to find work in the city, he became very despondent about his ability to survive. He knew that moving back to the rural areas would not help as there was even less employment available there. Though he had some extended family in the city, he missed his home and his mother in particular. She was in poor health, and he had hoped that he would be able to send her money, but now the situation felt hopeless. He began to feel more and more of a burden on the relatives he was staying with, and upon whom he was completely dependent as he had no form of income. Around this time, he began to have disturbing dreams from which he would wake up in the night, and then have difficulty falling asleep again. Going out to search for work began to feel like an increasing effort. Young men unable to find permanent or full-time employment would often wait by the side of the major road near the informal settlement where he was staying in the hope that they would be recruited to undertake manual labour for a day. Though he had found piecework in this way a few times, he found himself less and less able to join the group of other young men to wait for work. He began staying home more.

Mr Jaxa's great-aunt, with whom he was staying, was receiving an old age pension, which was effectively the only income for a household of eight people. Mr Jaxa's sombre presence inside all day became increasingly irritating to her, and she began chiding him more and more for not being a proper man who could earn a living. This was especially hurtful to Mr Jaxa. For a variety of reasons, including lack of money and his father having died when he was a child, Mr Jaxa had not yet undergone the circumcision process which would mark his entry into proper manhood. He felt angry with his great-aunt, and though he felt it wrong to do so, he became irritable and argued with her a great deal. His body began to feel tired and weak (from lack of physical exercise, he thought) and he began sleeping as much as he could during the day just to escape his situation. He began to take long walks to improve his strength but did not want to converse with people he met along the way. He would avoid them or deal with them abruptly. His great-aunt began complaining about him to neighbours, and told them she feared he might be bewitched. A sympathetic neighbour tried to befriend him and took him to a tavern one evening. There Mr Jaxa, who was unaccustomed to drinking alcohol, became intoxicated, and got involved in a loud argument with another patron who, with his friends, was taunting Mr Jaxa for his wandering around apparently aimlessly and for avoiding others. The possibly of Mr Jaxa's being bewitched was mentioned, and Mr Jaxa became very angry and threatened physical violence. A policeman who happened to be at the tavern intervened and removed Mr Jaxa from the tavern, fearing more for Mr Jaxa's safety than for that of the man he was arguing with. Having heard something about Mr Jaxa's plight, and about the allegation that Mr Jaxa was bewitched, the policeman thought it best not to take Mr Jaxa home. Having taken disruptive people with unusual behaviour to the casualty unit of the local general hospital before, the policeman did the same with Mr Jaxa.

After a long wait in a busy casualty unit, Mr Jaxa was seen by the doctor on duty. He was given a very brief opportunity to tell his story, which he did, mentioning his difficulties finding employment, his arguments with his great-aunt, his feelings of weakness and tiredness, and his general level of irritability. The doctor conducted a brief physical examination (partly to rule out a physical cause for Mr Jaxa's problems) and referred Mr Jaxa to the psychiatric casualty unit of the same hospital.

By the time Mr Jaxa arrived at psychiatric casualty, it was in the early hours of the morning. He was tired and feeling the after-effects of the alcohol. The doctor on duty was on call but not present. The professional nurse decided the best that could be done for Mr Jaxa would be to let him sleep off the alcohol and see the doctor in the morning.

The psychiatric registrar who saw Mr Jaxa the following morning was aware of the pressures on the casualty unit at night, and he also had had experience of patients who were seen as 'psychiatric' being treated cursorily in the general casualty unit. He therefore conducted another careful physical examination, and asked many questions about Mr Jaxa's state of physical health. He was not sure whether to believe Mr Jaxa when he said he was not a habitual drinker, and given the possibility of alcohol abuse and Mr Jaxa's being very thin, he prescribed vitamin tablets. For a full assessment and treatment plan, he referred Mr Jaxa to the admission unit of the nearby psychiatric hospital.

Mr Jaxa was taken to the psychiatric hospital by ambulance. On admission, he was seen by another psychiatric registrar, who took a brief history, checked on parts of the physical examination undertaken by her colleague at the psychiatric casualty unit, and took blood from Mr Jaxa as she wished to have an indication, amongst other things, of the possibility of sexually-transmitted disease (through a VDRL test), and thyroid functioning. Mr Jaxa was then referred to a clinical psychologist, for a full psychiatric assessment.

In response to the first question asked by the clinical psychologist – that of why Mr Jaxa was in hospital – he replied that he had many aches and pains, and problems with listlessness. On further questioning, Mr Jaxa also spoke about his irritability and feelings of hopelessness, his great-aunt's accusations of bewitchment, and his concerns about his not having been circumcised. He was able to give a good and coherent account of himself and his problems.

When the psychologist presented the case of Mr Jaxa at the case conference the following day, she mentioned that Mr Jaxa presented a clear case of cultural overlay on psychiatric illness. He was somatizing, and there were features in the history concerning bewitchment and cultural rituals. This seemed to be a case of masked depression and anxiety.

The outline of much of Mr Jaxa's story is a very familiar one in many parts of the world. Increasing joblessness and poverty are associated with massive migration to cities where, all too often, the promise of good housing, employment, and an income proves to be an illusion. The health and mental health impact of urbanization is difficult to measure, but research is beginning to document the challenges urbanization poses for health and social service workers (Desjarlais et al., 1995; Harpham & Blue, 1995; Harpham & Tanner, 1995; Yach et al., 1990). What is unusual about Mr Jaxa is that he has come to the attention of an inpatient psychiatric facility, especially as he has not gone through many of the stages of seeking help which we have discussed in Chapter 4 (cf. Goldberg & Huxley, 1992), and his behaviour was not particularly dramatic or socially disruptive.

The psychologist seeing Mr Jaxa had put together three things about what he had told her, to form what was, to her, a reasonably coherent 'cultural' picture. These three things were:

1 Mr Jaxa's first complaint to her was about physical symptoms.
2 The possibility of bewitchment was mentioned.
3 Mr Jaxa had not yet undergone circumcision, as was customary.

From her clinical experience, and from her reading of the local literature (see Swartz, 1986, 1987b for a review), the psychologist made sense of Mr Jaxa's manner of presentation as a 'cultural' one. There are many ways we can discuss this conclusion, but of interest to this chapter is the question of Mr Jaxa's 'somatizing' and what that means.

There are many different and competing definitions of somatization in the literature, but to introduce the topic here, I shall mention two easily accessible and contrasting views:

[S]omatization...[is]...the cultural patterning of psychological disorders into a 'language of distress' of mainly physical symptoms and signs. (Helman, 1994: 267)

Somatization...[is]...the presentation of personal and interpersonal distress in an idiom of physical complaints together with a coping pattern of medical help-seeking. (Kleinman, 1986: 51)

At first reading, these two definitions may seem substantially the same, but there are also crucial differences. According to Helman's definition, psychological disorders are *patterned* into a somatic or physical form. This implies that the basic condition is psychological, but there is a process whereby psychological experience changes into somatic experience. Kleinman's definition, by contrast, does not use the term 'psychological' at all, referring instead to 'distress', and speaking about *presentation* of an *idiom* of physical complaints, and a pattern of medical help-seeking. Kleinman does not necessarily see distress as primarily psychological, being transformed into something somatic. Another feature of his definition is that it makes explicit what he sees as what can be termed the *performative* nature of somatization. Instead of being viewed as purely an internal process, somatization can also be looked at as a means of conducting social interaction. Somatization can be seen as a strategy (not necessarily conscious) for getting help. In later work, Kleinman's emphasis has shifted even further from the idea of somatization as a particular, and special, idiom of distress. Discussing his work on illness and healing in China, he writes:

> Somatization seems normative and often normal; it is not so much a substitution for something more basic as it is a basic way of being-in-the-world. (Kleinman, 1995b:9)

Throughout the world, *including* the Western world, there is evidence that using the body to speak of and experience distress is in fact more common than experiencing distress and anxiety purely in psychological terms (Kleinman, 1986). A study examining the paths of patients to psychiatric care in eleven countries found that somatic problems were the most common manner of presentation, and that somatic complaints, as a way of presenting problems, were no more frequently seen in Third World than in other contexts (Gater et al., 1991). Similarly, Abas et al. (1995) found little difference in levels of somatization in primary care in Chile from those found in Britain – somatic presentations are common in both places. Why, then, is somatization so often treated as a problematic and foreign phenomenon?

Lock and Scheper-Hughes (1990) provide us with clues to the answer through the following story:

> We are reminded of a presentation that concerned the case of a middle-aged woman suffering from chronic and debilitating headaches. In halting sentences the patient explained before the large class of first-year medical students that her husband was an alcoholic who occasionally beat her, that she had been virtually housebound for the past five years looking after her senile and incontinent mother-in-law, and that she worried constantly about her teenage son, who was flunking out of high school. Although the woman's story elicited considerable sympathy from the students, one young woman finally interrupted the professor to demand, 'But what is the real cause of the headaches?' (Lock & Scheper-Hughes, 1990: 51)

Lock and Scheper-Hughes argue that the belief that the only 'real' thing is that which is physical has a long history in biomedicine, going back to Aristotle and Hippocrates, with the influence of Descartes in the seventeenth century being central. They show how uncomfortable health practitioners are when patients experience pain for which there is no obvious diagnosable physical cause. If a physical basis for this pain cannot be found, then within biomedicine it may be convenient to search for the 'reality' of the pain elsewhere – in the psychological realm. This enables us to speak of some physical pain as 'really' psychological in nature, and to think of somatization as a transformation of the 'psychological' reality into a physical form.

We have seen in the previous chapter how easy it is to place at the centre of our understanding our own views on how people operate. Leff (1988), for example, places the psychiatrist's knowledge at the forefront of people's own experiences of psychological difficulties. Similarly, if we take a narrowly physicalist understanding of the body – the understanding which has been so successful for biomedicine – as the ideal, then we rapidly reach a point where the bodily experience of distress comes to be seen as both somehow incorrect and unsophisticated. Tyrer (1982, quoted by Abas et al., 1995: 234), for example, makes the following bald evolutionist claim:

> [A]s a general rule, the more developed a society and the more intelligent its members, the greater the psychological component of anxiety symptoms ... Symptoms of free-floating anxiety are relatively uncommon in developing countries ... because of this tendency towards somatic emphasis. (Tyrer, 1982: 64)

Abas et al. comment: 'Such statements are remarkable in many respects, including the lack of reference to empirical data' (Abas et al., 1995: 234). The fact that the statement appeared in a standard handbook on mood disorders without, as Abas et al. point out, documented empirical evidence given, provides us with an indication of the degree to which it is commonly accepted that somatic presentation of distress is an 'unsophisticated' phenomenon associated with 'less developed' societies. What is at issue here, to some extent, is not whether there are different rates of somatization around the world, but the ways in which Western professionals' own cultural ideas about somatization interact with, and are influenced by, more general beliefs about race, culture, and sophistication (cf. Swartz, 1991b).

The history of professional constructions of psychological disorder in the Western world until recently tended to support an evolutionary view of a movement away from somatization as a way of experiencing distress towards a more psychological idiom. Neurasthenia, for example, was once thought to be common in the West, but is now seen as rare. Neurasthenia was defined in the 1920s as 'a condition of weakness or exhaustion of the nervous system, giving rise to various forms of mental and bodily inefficiency. The term covers an ill-defined, motley group of symptoms, which may be either general and the expression of derangement of the entire system, or local, limited to certain organs; hence the terms cerebral, spinal, cardiac, and gastric neurasthenia' (Pickering, 1974, as quoted by Kleinman, 1980: 129). Neurasthenia has fallen from use as a diagnostic category in the West, and is mentioned in the DSM-IV only in sections referring to specific cultural manifestations of mental disorder. By contrast, the diagnosis is common in China

(Kleinman, 1980, 1986). Similarly, Leff (1988) has shown how the diagnosis of hysteria – which often involves the use of the body to express distress – has become less and less common in the West.

The emergence of chronic fatigue syndrome as a phenomenon attracting considerable attention has helped raise questions about an evolutionist view of somatization. Chronic fatigue syndrome has reached prominence precisely because many of the sufferers from it are successful, middle-class Westerners. Chronic fatigue appears in the DSM-IV as 'undifferentiated somatoform disorder', but there is considerable debate as to the causes and nature of chronic fatigue syndrome (Hickie et al., 1995; Lawrie & Pelosi, 1995; Shanks & Ho-Yen, 1995; Sharpe et al., 1996; Surawy et al., 1995). What is clear is that the symptom profile greatly resembles that of neurasthenia, to the extent that it has been suggested that the terms may be effectively interchangeable (cf. Wessely, 1990). As we have seen with our discussion of depression in the previous chapter, then, an evolutionist view of somatization does not go very far in explaining the phenomenon.

Refining our ideas about somatization

How, then, do we explain somatization? In some respects, this is not a useful question. If somatization is common, and indeed normative in very many contexts throughout the world, then perhaps it would be more useful for us to ask how we explain 'psychologization' – the process whereby we come to see distress as primarily psychological or emotional in nature and presentation. Part of the answer to this lies in the cultural construction of the body and mind as separate and non-overlapping entities. If we view somatization simply as a 'defence mechanism', then we are privileging a psychological way of seeing the world, and losing much of the meaning that somatic expressions of distress can communicate.

Following Kirmayer's (1988, 1993) approach to somatization, Lewis-Fernández and Kleinman (1995) discuss an understanding of somatization which does not simply reduce it to a single mechanism of defence or a syndrome. In thinking about somatization, we need to consider it as a language, a way of seeing the world, and as a way of negotiating with the world. Lewis-Fernández and Kleinman (1995: 436) describe somatization as a 'way of engaging the world that translates meanings and social problems into individual processes of attention and communication'. Somatization is not necessarily a feature of illness at all, but simply a way of experiencing and engaging with the world.

Looking at somatization in this way allows us to consider different forms of somatization, and to understand their meaning in more depth. Kirmayer and Robbins describe three forms of somatization amongst patients in primary health care, and show that there is very little overlap between them. These three forms of somatization are:

a high levels of medically unexplained symptom reporting in multiple physiological systems ...
b levels of somatic preoccupation or illness worry beyond what is expected for demonstrable physical disease ...
c the predominantly or exclusively somatic clinical presentation of psychiatric disorder, most commonly depression and anxiety ... (Kirmayer & Robbins, 1991: 647).

The authors term patients in the first group *functional somatizers*, the second group *hypochondriacal somatizers*, and the third group *presenting somatizers*. In its extreme form, functional somatization can reach the level of severity where it meets the criteria for DSM-IV somatization disorder, which are as follows:

Diagnostic criteria for 300.81 Somatization Disorder
A A history of many physical complaints beginning before age 30 years that occur over a period of several years and result in treatment being sought or significant impairment in social, occupational, or other important areas of functioning.

B Each of the following criteria must have been met, with individual symptoms occurring at any time during the course of the disturbance:

1 four pain symptoms: a history of pain related to at least four different sites or functions (e.g., head, abdomen, back, joints, extremities, chest, rectum, during menstruation, during sexual intercourse, or during urination)

2 two gastrointestinal symptoms: a history of at least two gastrointestinal symptoms other than pain (e.g., nausea, bloating, vomiting other than during pregnancy, diarrhea, or intolerance of several different foods)

3 one sexual symptom: a history of at least one sexual or reproductive symptom other than pain (e.g., sexual indifference, erectile or ejaculatory dysfunction, irregular menses, excessive menstrual bleeding, vomiting throughout pregnancy)

4 one pseudoneurological symptom: a history of at least one symptom or deficit suggesting a neurological condition not limited to pain (conversion symptoms such as impaired coordination or balance, paralysis or localized weakness, difficulty swallowing or lump in throat, aphonia, urinary retention, hallucinations, loss of touch or pain sensation, double vision, blindness, deafness, seizures; dissociative symptoms such as amnesia; or loss of consciousness other than fainting)

C Either (1) or (2):

1 after appropriate investigation, each of the symptoms in Criterion B cannot be fully explained by a known general medical condition or the direct effects of a substance (e.g., a drug of abuse, a medication)

2 when there is a related general medical condition, the physical complaints or resulting social or occupational impairment are in excess of what would be expected from the history, physical examination, or laboratory findings

D The symptoms are not intentionally feigned or produced (as in Factitious Disorder or Malingering). (DSM-IV, 1994: 449-450)

According to Kirmayer and Robbins (1991: 654), 'functional somatizers ... are often neither depressed nor exceptionally worried about their health'. This last factor contrasts with hypochondriacal soma-tizers, who are preoccupied with their health and tend to be distressed by this preoccupation. This picture differs also from somatic pre-senters who 'often display neither high levels of functional sympto-matology nor hypochondriacal worry and may simply be suffering from the well-described somatic concomitants of depression or anxiety, including vegetative symptoms and pain. These patients attribute their complaints to physical rather than psychological causes, with varying degrees of certainty or conviction. Most are quite willing to consider the psychosocial dimensions of their problems with minimal prompting' (Kirmayer & Robbins, 1991: 654).

Thinking about somatization in Africa

Although the Kirmayer and Robbins study was conducted in Canada, a very different cultural context from southern Africa, it is very useful conceptually in that it helps us be more specific in what we are saying about somatization in this part of the world. Studies of somatization in Africa tend not to be specific about what aspects are being invest-igated, but tend to focus on the question of somatic presenters rather than on the other two types (Abas et al., 1995; Petersen & Parekh, 1996; Peltzer, 1995; Thom et al., 1993). For example, Miller et al. (1991) found that 45 per cent of people presenting at primary health care facil-ities in a village in the Western Cape scored above the cut-off on a measure of psychiatric morbidity. Though the study was method-ologically unsophisticated, a follow-up qualitative study of high scorers (Rogers, 1992) suggests that a psychologically informed approach to diagnosis and management in these cases would be helpful (cf. Swartz & Miller, 1992a).

Studying somatization in primary health care can be challenging methodologically. In a study of outpatients attending a clinic in KwaZulu/Natal, for example, Petersen and Parekh (1996) found that roughly half of the patients in this volunteer sample scored above the cut-off on a screening test for psychiatric morbidity (the screen used was the Self-Reporting Questionnaire, or SRQ; Beusenberg & Orley, 1994; Harding et al., 1980). When the SRQ results were factor analysed, the two major factors found were *neurasthenia* – a mixture of anxiety, depressive, and physical complaints – and *somatic symptoms*. The authors conclude that 'in relation to the form of minor psychiatric symptoms, there is a prominence of somatic and neurasthenia symptoms' (Petersen & Parekh, 1996: 72). At first reading, this makes sense, but there may be a problem with the reasoning given. To show how important it is to think clearly about somatization, it is worth going through the logic of their argument step by step:

1 Based on other research both internationally and in southern Africa, the authors set out to find out about minor psychiatric disorders in primary health care.
2 They administer the SRQ to a volunteer sample at a clinic.
3 They find that roughly half of these volunteers score over the cut-off on the SRQ.
4 Factor analysis of the SRQ results reveals the following two main factors:
   Neurasthenia
   Items loading on this factor, in order of strength of the load: *Are you easily tired?; Do you find it difficult to make decisions?; Do you feel unhappy?*.
   Somatic symptoms
   Items loading on this factor, in order of strength of the load: *Is your appetite poor? ; Do you sleep badly?; Is your digestion poor?; Do you often have headaches?*.
5 On the basis of this, they conclude that 'in relation to the form of minor psychiatric symptoms, there is a prominence of somatic and neurasthenia symptoms'. (Petersen & Parekh, 1996: 72)

If we explore the symptoms which load on to the first two factors, at least five of the seven are arguably somatic symptoms (tiredness, headaches, poor appetite, poor digestion, poor sleeping), with two more 'psychological' in nature (unhappiness, impaired decision-making). But what does this mean? The patients, as we have seen, are all attending a primary health care clinic. Some of them may well be suffering from physical disorders which have as their symptoms many of those loading on the two major factors. Gastroenteritis, for example, could easily present with tiredness, headaches, poor appetite and digestion, difficulties sleeping, and even unhappiness. Without knowing the full picture of answers to all the SRQ questions, we cannot be sure what Petersen and Parekh (1996) have found, but the symptoms which are discussed do not necessarily lead to a conclusion that we are dealing here with a somatic presentation of anxiety and depression.

Through methods other than this, and through the collection of other data, Petersen and Parekh (1996) and their colleagues (Petersen et al., 1996) are able to make a convincing argument for the importance of dealing with psychological issues in primary health care, but what has happened around this small aspect of their work is instructive. The SRQ contains many 'somatic' items precisely because of the mass of work all over the world which suggests that somatic presentation of personal distress is important. But somatic conditions *also* present with somatic features (obviously), as well as psychological features. To conclude that items, simply because they are in the SRQ, must be seen as psychiatric symptoms is clearly premature. Other information – on the absence of demonstrable physical pathology, for example – would be necessary. The question of physical and psychological complaints occurring together also needs to be considered (Kisely & Goldberg, 1996).

There can be no question of the importance of recognizing that in primary health care a proportion of people who first present with somatic features will, on careful assessment, be found to be more properly thought of as anxious and/or depressed. Mental health practitioners have an important role to play in bringing this important clinical information to the attention of primary health care personnel. Equally important, though, is the need to make sure that adequate physical care is not abandoned. Patients who present atypically, or who are simply unusually anxious people, may easily be stigmatized as 'psychological cases' or malingerers – to the detriment of adequate primary health care.

There is some irony in this argument. People concerned to bring the phenomenon of somatization to the attention of those who have tended in the past to reduce everything to the biological level and have dismissed somatization as not 'real', may be in some danger themselves of entering into a reductionism of another kind. This reductionism consists of viewing everything as psychogenic, and of seeing the somatic as not 'real' in some cases. This 'psychological reductionism' is as problematic as viewing only the demonstrably somatic as real (cf. Kleinman & Kleinman, 1991). This can become a problem for clinicians as opposed to a matter relevant only to academic discussion. This is partly because stigma is interwoven so tightly both with attributions of somatization and with psychological problems in general. To many people, including, unfortunately, many clinicians, having psychological problems is something to be ashamed of. When concerned mental health professionals enter the realm of primary health care and inform practitioners about somatic presentation of depression and anxiety, they are not only giving potentially clinically useful information. They are also potentially adding to some patients the stigmatized label of 'psychological case'. Later in this book we will see some examples of how profoundly this type of labelling can affect the way patients are treated – and not only for the better. So it is essential that we are both accurate about somatic presentation when it is present and prepared for reactions by professionals to this information. Over-labelling somatization is not helpful. Because, as we have seen, the view is widely held that somatization is a feature of 'less sophisticated' societies, special care needs to be taken that the perception does not arise that somatization – like many other ills – is always and exclusively a problem of stigmatized and relatively powerless groups. Aspects of this theme will be returned to in the following chapter.

An example of how labelling about somatization and psychological involvement in somatic presentation raises complex questions can be seen from an experience I had some years ago. My colleagues and I (Miller et al., 1991) were interested in psychological factors in primary health care in a small village. In preparation for our study we met informally with primary health care personnel serving the area. They told us that emotional problems presenting as physical complaints were very common. One of the practitioners remarked that '95 per cent' of his patients did not have an organic disorder. We designed a simple study to explore this. Over a week, we assessed all patients at primary health care settings in the area using the General Health Questionnaire (GHQ; Goldberg, 1972, 1978; Goldberg & Hillier, 1979). We also asked practitioners independently to fill out a form with the question 'To what extent do you think psychological or stress factors have contributed to the decision of the patient to come to the doctor today?'.

Even making allowance for exaggeration, the informal estimates of practitioners were very different from what we found. Only five individuals, out of a sample 159 patients (3.14 per cent), were rated by practitioners to have psychological factors accounting for a major part of or their entire decision to present at a primary health care service – a figure much lower than our assessment, using the GHQ. Without more detailed information on the practitioners' beliefs it is not possible to provide a full interpretation of this finding, but it is useful in the context of the present discussion to consider some possibilities. One of these is that when practitioners work in a busy, understaffed primary health care context, they remember those patients for whom they felt they could do very little, or whose manner of presentation does not fit neatly into recognizable organic symptom profiles, and they overestimate the number of such people that they see. It may also be that in describing their practice as dominated by somatization, which, without any training at the time, they found difficult to deal with, they were telling us about their own experience of their work as difficult. These are just two possibilities, both of which have bearing on how we should be thinking if we want to increase awareness of somatic presentation amongst primary health care personnel.

There is another important possible interpretation of our observations. It may be that what we term 'psychological' and what the practitioners understood by the term are different. The practitioner who estimated that 95 per cent of his patients did not have organic problems commented that 'most of them just want time off work'. (The issue of legitimacy regarding time off work is clearly also an important one for patients in poor communities, as we have seen from Mr Carolus's story at the beginning of the previous chapter). One might conclude that this 'wanting time off work' is not perceived by this practitioner to be a psychological factor. His disparaging tone of voice when making this comment suggests that giving it the label 'psychological', or speaking of stress, might mean giving the behaviour a status which requires attention and has some value, and he seems reluctant to do this (Swartz & Miller, 1992a).

In an interview, this same practitioner described the people of the village where he was working as 'without morals' and 'lazy'. It may be, then, that he viewed the somatic presentation of what he saw as reluctance to work as a moral issue. He was operating from the perspective of judging his patients' behaviour rather than attempting to understand it from their point of view. In this context, the label 'somatization' may come to be used not to help practitioners see the psychological component of their patients' behaviour but instead to label patients' behaviour. This label helps maintain a distance between patients and practitioners, especially where there are class, gender, and cultural differences between them. Patients can be viewed as 'unsophisticated', and also as morally suspect if they present their personal distress in somatic forms.

Clearly, this type of distancing and labelling of patients is exactly the opposite of what a culturally and psychologically informed approach to somatization is trying to do. It is very important therefore that any attempt to introduce an understanding of somatization into primary health care, and health care in general, should not overstate its case, and should anticipate the possibility of a degree of misunderstanding. In Chapter 1 of this book I argued that any understanding of culture and mental health must take account of the ways in which professionals understand these issues. The above example regarding somatization reinforces this view. In the following section we shall briefly explore this issue further.

Somatization: patient problem or practitioner construction?

This chapter opened with the story of Mr Jaxa. As a result of his life problems he entered the medical system and within a few days was presented at a case conference as 'somatizing'. This is a summary of his contact with professionals since his admission to the casualty unit of the general hospital:

1 He was given a physical examination by the doctor on duty in the general casualty unit.
2 He was transferred to psychiatric casualty where the professional nurse on duty arranged that he sleep over.
3 The psychiatric registrar who saw him the following morning conducted a thorough physical examination, and prescribed tablets.
4 He was taken by ambulance to a psychiatric hospital.
5 On admission he was examined by another doctor, who took blood.
6 He met the clinical psychologist in charge of the case, and the first thing that he told her was that he had aches and pains and listlessness.

Mr Jaxa has been through a process which has focused on physical examinations and blood tests. It has taken place in hospitals, where doctors and nurses were around. He has been in an ambulance. This has been appropriate biomedical care. It is also easy to imagine, though, that Mr Jaxa has gained the impression that what concerns the health system he was brought to for help is his physical well-being. His story on admission to the medical casualty unit was not primarily a medical one; by the time he reaches the clinical psychologist, he may have learned that a medical story is what is wanted. The fact that this is not the case may have more to do with the contradictory position of mental health care in the health system than with any lack of insight by Mr Jaxa. The entrance to the world of the mind, if we can describe the psychiatric facility in this way, has been through the world of the body – the world of aches, pains, and fatigue. If anything, it may be more accurate to say it is the health care system which engages in a process of somatizing of a kind, rather than Mr Jaxa. The health care system, for good reason, has presented itself to Mr Jaxa as interested in physical signs and symptoms, and has not, until the interview with the psychologist, laid as much stress on the psychological. It is therefore a misreading of the term 'somatization' to ascribe this to Mr Jaxa. Part of why this was done, as we have seen, is that Mr Jaxa also spoke about circumcision and bewitchment issues. Much of this chapter has shown, though, that there is a powerful myth amongst professionals that somatization is a feature of 'unsophisticated' people or people whom biomedicine has difficulty understanding. Somatization has become linked with other features which biomedicine may find culturally strange. To an extent, Mr Jaxa is becoming stereotyped. This is probably done out of the well-intentioned desire to provide culture-sensitive treatment to Mr Jaxa, but stereotyping is happening nonetheless.

Mr Jaxa's story (elicited retrospectively after these events) indicates that from the beginning of his difficulties, he experienced his problems in a mixture of interpersonal, psychological, and physical terms. There is a tradition within psychosomatic medicine of referring to patients with psychosomatic disorders as suffering from 'alexithymia' – having no words for feelings (Sifneos, 1973). Clearly, this does not adequately describe Mr Jaxa, who is able to speak about his feelings with little difficulty. A further potential problem with the somatization label for him is that professionals are not always clear on different meanings of the term, as shown by Kirmayer and Robbins (1991), and discussed earlier. It is never enough to describe a person as somatizing – one must say what one means about how the body is being used to experience and communicate distress. When professionals engage with this question in the particular contexts in which patients live and find themselves, they are far less likely to use 'somatization' simply as a label, and they are more likely to explore the meanings involved in patients' communicating with the body.

In my view, there is very little evidence to suggest that somatization (as a feature of patients) is a part of Mr Jaxa's presentation. It is more likely that the term is being used because of the clinician's desire to be sensitive to cultural issues. What, though, of Mr Carolus, whose story opened the previous chapter? His ongoing concern with his back pain is certainly suggestive of a pattern of using the body to experience and communicate distress. Once again, though, until and unless we are fully informed about the nature and appropriateness of the care that was and was not received after the accident, we cannot be sure whether our assumptions are accurate.

Part of the problem we face here is that if, as Kleinman (1995a: 9) suggests, 'somatization is a basic way of being-in-the-world', a way of living our lives rather than a specific symptom, syndrome, or strategy, then we cannot simply use somatization as a label. The challenge is not so much to find out who somatizes and who does not, but to incorporate an understanding of the meanings of somatization in all clinical work. This challenge is one which goes to the heart of biomedicine, as it requires engagement with the possibility that minds and bodies are not as separable as it would be convenient to maintain. We shall see in the following chapter how the phenomenon of 'nerves' raises these same issues for our thinking about culture and mental health, though in a slightly different way.

7

Nervous bodies, shattered minds

Elvira is a 53-year-old woman living in a small village in an old and ramshackle house with her husband, five sons, two daughters, daughter-in-law, and ten grandchildren. She would like her married son and his wife and five children to move out of the house, but they cannot find suitable accommodation. Only her husband, an unskilled worker, and one of the sons are employed. Elvira looks after the children during the day, and is also responsible for housework, commenting that 'when they come in, everything must be right – otherwise there's a problem'.

Elvira went to her primary care doctor because of an upset stomach and stomach pains. She reports that the doctor told her she had an 'infection' in her stomach, and also told her that 'stomach nerves' were responsible for the pain. He said she had eaten 'heavy meat' which she had not chewed properly as her bottom teeth had been extracted. She asked the doctor why she so often had headaches. According to Elvira, he took a blood sample from her, and informed her that her 'blood [pressure] was up'.

A week before going to the doctor, Elvira had woken up with a severe headache. She felt tired, weak, and shaky, and her legs felt lame. She lay on the bed for a day on account of the lameness in her legs. Initially her stomach felt full, thick, and bloated. Then the pain moved to the middle of her stomach, and she experienced a burning sensation. Her stomach became very painful and diarrhoea began. She could not eat. She told her daughter of the pain and discomfort, and her daughter gave her boiling water to drink together with a herbal remedy. Before going to the doctor, Elvira worried that her stomach pain was similar to that experienced by her niece, who had stayed with them six months previously. The niece had become ill with stomach pain, and within a short time had died in the hospital of stomach cancer.

In retrospect, Elvira feels that her 'high blood' problems were caused by 'the upset on the weekend, the grown children, and their drinking'. She had wanted to escape the home situation: 'Sometimes I feel I want to go out, to get away from the problems, the bustle in the house'. She reports that although she had been diagnosed as 'high blood' before, she had not experienced this as a problem prior to the weekend when she became ill. 'I never felt bad; only now that the children began with drinking problems, I get so upset'. As mother of the house, she feels she must make everything right: 'Everything has to be right because the drink says – I want this, I want that ... sometimes I am not good enough in their eyes. But now I don't want to tire myself out about it any more. I feel that my health is going down; I am the one who will suffer.'

Elvira reports that her illness is better since she went to the doctor and took the pills he prescribed, 'because the doctor's pills are very good'. At present she is taking 'stomach nerve pills, pain pills, calming pills, and medicine which works together with the pills'. She would like a tonic to get her appetite back – at times she does not eat for three days at a time, drinking only boiling water. After four days of taking the medication, the lameness disappeared and the headaches went away. She feels that if she had not consulted the doctor she would still be lying in pain, and would have had to stay in bed for a long time as she felt 'so exhausted'. Without treatment, she would have 'gone to ground'. She feels that if she does not go back to the doctor and take her medicine, the problem will recur, because 'stomach nerves is not something that goes away – if you come home and get upset, then you get nerves'. She feels that she may need additional medicine for her nerves.

She hopes that as a result of her nerves, her family will try to deal with their alcohol problems so that they won't affect her so much and so that she can 'get more calmness'. The family members know about her illness, and they are trying to be more considerate and to drink less, but when friends are there, they still drink. She comments that 'drink problems break up a house'. (Adapted from Rogers, 1992: 46-49)

The doctor's opinion about Elvira's complaints is unfortunately not available, but regardless of this, it is clear that for Elvira social and inter-personal difficulties are strongly tied up with experiences of the body. Elvira lives as a black ('coloured') South African in a small village (Mamre) in a situation of poverty and overcrowding. By virtue of her gender and age she is expected to keep the home together and look after the children. She receives little support from her family and is, arguably, abused by them. In her understanding, her illness is a conse-quence of her situation. The illness also gains her certain benefits, like being able to rest for a day, and gives her a way of addressing the alcohol abuse in the home (admittedly with limited success). From a narrowly biomedical perspective, Elvira's description of her illness and treatment may seem naïve and misinformed. If we take another approach, though, we can see that Elvira's formulation of illness in a psychosocial context bears much similarity to professional under-standings within the field of psychosomatic medicine.

In Rogers's (1992) study, of which Elvira's case is a part, she found that over half of an unselected group of people attending primary health care in a South African village reported that, either currently or in the past, they suffered from their nerves. Nerves were described in many ways, primarily as bodily disorders or pain. The stomach was the primary site for nerves, which was reported to consist of stomach pain and cramps; a feeling in the stomach similar to hunger; a stomach turning over; 'if something upsets me, my stomach gets sore'. Headaches could also be a feature of nerves, as could insomnia, poor appetite, restlessness, fatigue, and lameness in the legs. All these features tended to operate together, as in: 'If you are on your nerves, then you feel bad, your tummy works, you are restless, and you can't sleep'. Emotions were also seen to be part of nerves – tension, sadness and weepiness, anxiety, and feeling hysterical. Nerves was related by respondents to poor economic conditions, to worries, to bad feelings, and to interpersonal conflict.

A remarkable feature of Rogers's findings is that they echo findings in many other parts of the world – nerves has been described in Latin America, in Greece, in North America, in Ireland (Davis & Low, 1989), as well as in South Africa (Reynolds & Swartz, 1993; Swartz & Miller, 1992a, 1992b). Clearly, the mixture of emotional and physical experiences of nerves links it to neurasthenia, as discussed in the previous chapter, and neurasthenia is still an important diagnosis in China (Lee, 1996a). If nerves is so widespread, though, in what way should it be considered an object of cultural analysis? Jenkins and Valiente (1994) comment:

> Long-standing dualisms of the mind as cultural and the body as biological have often served to render the physical, sensational world of pangs, vapors, and twinges theoretically insignificant and largely absent from cultural-symbolic analysis. (Jenkins & Valiente, 1994: 164)

They argue further that there is a 'traditional dualist idea that the closer we come to the body the farther away we must be from culture' (Jenkins & Valiente, 1994: 164). Clearly, the story of Elvira, like many stories from other parts of the world (see, for example, Csordas, 1994; Finkler, 1991, 1994; Kleinman, 1986; Levy et al., 1987; Lock, 1990; Rubel et al., 1984; Scheper-Hughes, 1992), demonstrates the importance of a cultural understanding of a mixture of bodily and emotional experiences. Thinking about nerves as experienced both physically and emotionally helps us break away from having to decide whether an experience is primarily 'physical' or 'psychological'. Instead, we can begin to consider questions about how experiences are embodied (Finkler, 1989) in the context of people's lives and their interaction with healing systems.

As we have seen in the previous chapter, we cannot, in thinking about the body and the emotions, simply resort to 'somatization' as a label. We also cannot see concerns about the body, and the expression of distress through the body as a feature only of 'unsophisticated' people. On the contrary, the body as a site of interest has taken on extra significance in the contemporary (what some would refer to as the postmodern) world:

> The body, or embodied subject, is the object of seduction by advertising, interpellation by semiotically loaded commodities, torture by a broad spectrum of political regimes, bitter conflicts over reproductive rights and health care, struggles for the revaluation of alternate sexual identities, threats from new epidemic diseases, the object of new technologies permitting the alteration of physical attributes hitherto accepted as naturally determined, including cosmetic surgery, asexual and extra-bodily fertilization, multiple forms of intervention in the biological process of reproduction, the modification of genetic traits, and the artificial prolongation or curtailment of the span of life itself. In these and other ways, the body seems thrust into ever-increasing prominence of social conflicts and repressive controls, as well as some of the most liberating aspects of contemporary culture and social life. (Turner, 1994: 27)

In the history of medicine and psychiatry, furthermore, there has long been a concern with whether madness can be detected through the image of the body, and with the AIDS epidemic there is renewed interest in the image of the body as both seductive and dangerous, pure and diseased (Gilman, 1995). In short, the body is currently being seen as more profoundly social and cultural than ever before (Scheper-Hughes & Lock, 1987). Thus, when Lock speaks of 'the way in which the physical body is the only available means for expressing dissent by people in structurally powerless situations' (Lock, 1989: 82), it must not be assumed that use of the body as a mode of expression is confined only to those in 'structurally powerless situations'. On the contrary, the use of the body – and the problem of nerves – needs to be understood in the context of a view of the world which recognizes the political realities which create an environment within which suffering from nerves becomes a representation, in part, of social forces of oppression. Reviewing a series of articles on nerves in various settings,

Lock (1989) comments that each of the groups of nerves-sufferers discussed

> is clearly disadvantaged, their traditional culture fractured and fragmented so that the seamless web of culture has been ripped open, and where once harmony and emotional control were valued, now anger and rage simmer perpetually inside the body and erupt at every provocation into '*ataques de nervios*' or '*nevra*'. This is the non-verbal language of the powerless… (Lock, 1989: 85)

For Lock, then, the study of nerves becomes the study not of the powerless or the 'unsophisticated', but the study of relationships of power in themselves, as well as the study of what have been termed 'weapons of the weak' (Scott, 1985; Turner, 1969). It will be interesting to see how this approach holds up in looking at nerves in the southern African context.

I first became interested in nerves through a different route from that taken by the many anthropologists who have studied the phenomenon. In general, anthropological accounts at the time emphasized the ways in which nerves is used as a term by lay people as an idiom of distress, as a way of interacting with and attempting to gain some control over the world (as in the case of Elvira), and as a way of embodying experience (Davis, 1989b; Davis & Guarnaccia, 1989; Dunk, 1989; Guarnaccia, DeLaCancela et al., 1989; Guarnaccia & Farias, 1988; Guarnaccia, Rubio-Stipec et al., 1989; Lock, 1989; Low, 1985; Nations et al., 1988). Less frequently, there were also detailed discussions of professionals' responses to nerves as a folk illness (Finkler, 1991; Low, 1988), and of professional traditions which had apparently contributed to nerves being a common phenomenon (Davis, 1989a; Davis & Whitten, 1988; Low, 1988). Although I had known that Xhosa-speaking people sometimes use the term *iinerves* as a loan word from English (Swartz et al., 1985), I developed an interest in nerves only after I was asked to join the Mamre Community Health Project. I first heard the term nerves not from the people of Mamre, but from researchers from outside the community trying to develop an understanding of psychiatric disorder in that community. In discussing my and my colleagues' involvement in this project, I hope to show some of the issues the phenomenon of nerves highlights for southern Africans interested in mental heath issues.

Nerves in the Mamre Community Health Project

The Mamre Community Health Project (MCHP) was started in the mid-1980s as a public health research initiative emphasizing the development of research skills, community participation, and interventions to improve the health of the people of Mamre (Katzenellenbogen et al., 1988, 1995, 1997). Mamre is situated approximately 50 kilometres from Cape Town, the inhabitants (roughly 5 000 in number) were classified 'coloured' under the apartheid system, and are largely working-class. The project was run by a multidisciplinary research team which included medical practitioners, epidemiologists, statisticians and nurses, as well as community members, and the Mamre Community Health Programme, under community control, was still operating there at the time of writing. In 1986, the MCHP undertook as its first task the assessment of ill health (including psychiatric illness) in Mamre. A community-wide household health survey was thus designed. The term 'psychiatric illness' was thought to be inaccessible to the respondents, and therefore the term *senuwees* (Afrikaans for nerves) was substituted. This is a term which is in general use in the Mamre community and was assumed to be a folk category roughly corresponding to the professional category of psychiatric illness.

In the pilot phase of the household health survey conducted in the nearby village of Pella, however, it emerged that large numbers of people, and women especially, when questioned, were identifying themselves as having suffered from nerves. This suggested that respondents were interpreting nerves more broadly than the researchers had intended. In order to focus more specifically on psychiatric disorder, the research team modified the nerves question to cover only hospital or outpatient treatment for nerves. This more specific question resulted in a prevalence of 2.92 per cent, with an approximately three to one ratio of women to men (Hoffman et al., 1988). Because of the high prevalence of nerves, particularly before the methods were refined to exclude persons who believed they suffered from nerves but had not been treated for nerves, I was asked to join the project team to study nerves further. Full details of the way the work was tackled are given in Swartz & Miller (1992a); I will focus here on specific questions surrounding nerves.

Nerves and psychiatric disorder

The research team had clearly decided to use 'nerves' to mean mental disorder. One of the first questions to be asked is whether this was in fact valid. The literature on nerves in other parts of the world suggests that nerves and mental illness are not synonymous. Much of the literature clearly distinguishes between nerves and mental illness (Davis, 1989b; Davis & Guarnaccia, 1989; Davis & Whitten, 1988; Guarnaccia et al., 1989; Jenkins, 1988; Low, 1985; Nations et al., 1985, 1988). Davis and Whitten (1988) do acknowledge, however, that nerves and mental illness are related in some way in Newfoundland: they seem to suggest that nerves and mental illness lie on a continuum, although there is disagreement amongst villagers 'as to what constitutes the limits of "just nerves" and the beginning of mental illness'. Jenkins (1988), unlike most other researchers, argues that nerves is used by Mexican-Americans in relation to schizophrenia. *Nervios* was the most common term used by Mexican-American relatives of schizophrenic patients to describe their relatives' problem.

If the nerves category subsumes psychiatric disorder in Mamre, one would anticipate that many known psychiatric patients we interviewed would claim to suffer from nerves. Many patients described their experiences of psychiatric illness in terms of problems with their nerves. There were several ways of doing this, and these differed in the degree to which the nerves category overlapped with the psychiatric illness category.

For some, nerves was a factor causing the illness. For example, Ms A, in describing her husband's acute psychotic episode, described his bizarre behaviour and somatic experiences, claiming that these had 'worked on his nerves'. His illness, however, was not nerves, but 'veins calcified in the head'.

Others understood nerves to be a substantial part of the illness, but some distinction between nerves and the illness seemed nonetheless to be made. In describing her schizophrenic illness, particularly the aetiology and onset of the illness, Ms B said (quotations are taken from different parts of the interview):

> [T]hey said that my nerves, because I was so clever, worked too fast; I was 15 when I had a nervous collapse. I was young. The brain gave in, almost gave in. I was off my head, I heard voices ... [which said] I must hurt my mother ... Then I said they are all devils, they want to bewitch me ... Then I talk confused; my nerves were too bad, I was too empty, then they had to give me treatment at Stikland [a psychiatric hospital].

She spontaneously and frequently talks about her nerves and her (psychotic) behaviour and experiences, implicitly linking them very closely. However, when asked what nerves means she says: 'You're anxious and you're scared'. In another comment she again reveals her 'definition' of nerves: 'Further I'm also on my nerves, also very shaky, anxious. Anxious, shaky and anxious'. In other words, although there is a considerable overlap between nerves and her illness, Ms B does not see the two as entirely synonymous.

A majority of patients and relatives use the terms nerves or nervous collapse (*senuwees, senuweesinstorting, senuweesineenstorting*) as the term to describe the mental illness experience. When Ms C was asked whether or not she was employed, she explained that she was unemployed, but had worked until the nervous collapse began. Ms D replied to a question about treatment by saying that she was 'under treatment for nerves', as did Mr E, who said he 'takes pills for nerves'. When Mr F was asked whether he had any health problems, he answered affirmatively, saying he suffered from 'tension'; when asked what he calls his problem, he replied 'nervous collapse'. The F family, throughout the interview, seemed to use the terms tension, nerves, and nervous collapse interchangeably, as did others (for example, the B family). They also mentioned stomach nerves, which was experienced by Mr F's stepmother.

Despite the frequent connection of nerves with behaviour associated with psychiatric illness, some people clearly differentiated between nerves and madness. Ms A said that her husband's behaviour was 'almost like a mad person'. She seemed to be implicitly distinguishing between his experience and madness. Ms C (diagnosed as suffering from hypomania and schizophrenia), in describing her admission to a psychiatric hospital, said: 'that's not a place that I belong, because all the people there are confused, their eyes are wild and they make you like that'. This reluctance to associate nerves and madness may be due to the stigma associated with madness. It may be that nerves stands for signs defined by clinicians as psychiatric, and that like psychiatrically trained professionals, our respondents avoid the term madness.

Not all psychiatric patients believed that they suffered from their nerves. It is not entirely clear whether this is because they see nerves as different from what they do suffer from (a psychiatric or other category different from nerves) or whether they would deny suffering from any illness – whether psychiatric or nerves. Evidence in support of the first possibility comes from Mr B who said: 'I have no problems with my nerves. It's just the voices, soft (*fyn*) little voices that I still hear'. At least some of the psychiatric patients we interviewed denied any emotional, psychiatric, or nerves illness at all, consistently objecting to the constructions others had placed on their behaviour.

In summary, it appears that unlike most other descriptions of nerves in the literature, nerves in Mamre cannot be easily separated from mental illness. A large majority of patients and relatives use the term nerves when talking about their experiences of psychiatric illness, although the degree to which nerves and mental illness coincide, varies. The fact, however, that approximately half of the psychiatric patients and half of the *relatives* of psychiatric patients admit to being nerves-sufferers suggests that nerves does not simply refer to psychiatric illness.

Nerves sufferers and primary care practitioners talk about nerves

In order to develop a more sophisticated qualitative understanding of nerves, Reynolds (1990) interviewed a small sample of nerves sufferers about their condition. He also questioned a representative from each of the medical practices operating in Mamre (this includes district surgeons and panel doctors) about their approach to nerves and its management. This second section of his research is considered in Reynolds and Swartz (1993).

As might be expected, all the seven nerves sufferers interviewed in depth by Reynolds related the condition to psychosocial stressors including poverty and violence and drug and alcohol abuse in the home. Respondents distinguished between *kopsenuwees* ('head nerves') characterized by headaches or a general feeling of malaise, and *maagsenuwees* ('stomach nerves') which involved a hollow feeling in the stomach or gastrointestinal complaints including, apparently, ulcers. *Hartsenuwees* ('heart nerves') apparently also occurs. A surprising finding was that the majority of respondents had first labelled themselves as having nerves when they had been told by medical practitioners that they had the condition. This finding flew in the face of our assumption that nerves was generally a condition which people brought to the doctor and which doctors then transformed into more formal disease categories.

Chapter 1 stressed the importance of the recognition of explanatory models in clinical practice. It is possible that doctors in Mamre were using the term 'nerves' in the process of negotiating with patients. The question of negotiation of models, however, is far from simple. Explanatory models, popular and professional, are not necessarily categorically separate or opposed (Swartz, 1987a), as we have seen in Chapter 4. Professionals themselves are not immune from cultural influence, and they hold a range of cultural beliefs which affect their interpretation and use of professional models. They bring the influence of their own, non-formal, socialization to their professional practice (Gilbert & Mulkay, 1984), possibly particularly so in the case of health professionals, who deal with many issues which are, at some level, inherently moral (Hahn & Gaines, 1985). From a practical point of view, furthermore, it is all very well to speak of 'negotiation' but this does not give clinicians a blueprint of how to act. With these issues in mind, Reynolds interviewed the clinicians in Mamre, and an incident which occurred during data collection amplified for us the probable construction of nerves in the clinical context.

Here is one story which told us a great deal about nerves. A medical practitioner (Dr 1) told the interviewer that where people complain spontaneously of nerves, the complaints are usually located in the stomach – people will complain of *maag wat krap* ('upset stomach') or *hol kol op die maag* ('hollow feeling in the stomach'). He sees these problems as gastric complaints related to underlying stressors.

Dr 1 uses these terms even when patients do not bring them spontaneously to the consultation, and especially when dealing with patients whom he believes to be somatizing. He operates under the assumption that even if patients do not understand these words, they would at least have heard of them. Where further explanation is required, a vague medical explanation is given; according to Dr 1 there is no point in being too technical. He believes it is important for patients to be able to communicate to others what their problems are in terms that those people will understand. It is also important to give a consistent explanation to the patient; the use of the term 'nerves' is an easy way of doing this. Given his approach to the use of the term 'nerves', then, Dr 1 would tell a patient with a gastric ulcer, for example, that the problem is *maagsenuwees* ('stomach nerves').

A patient who had been given the diagnosis of *maagsenuwees* by Dr 1 reported that she had received white medicine for the condition, but that a friend who had been prescribed the same medication by another practitioner had been diagnosed as having a stomach ulcer. She asked the interviewer to explain why the same medicine had been prescribed for two different conditions – *maagsenuwees* on the one hand, and stomach ulcer on the other. Clearly, she did not ascribe different status to the 'folk' and 'professional' labels – she saw the labels as both having come from professionals and as necessarily designating different conditions.

From this example we can see that Dr 1's choice to speak about nerves in order to make clinical communication easier was not interpreted in this way by the patient. She viewed the term *maag-senuwees* as a professional diagnosis. This is not surprising in the light of Dr 1's position as a professional; it is not unlikely that many patients would view everything said by doctors as professional knowledge. Some support for the view that Dr 1's patients, and other Mamre residents, may regard nerves as a professional rather than a folk term comes from our finding that most patients we interviewed said that doctors were the first people to tell them that they suffered from their nerves.

A substantial proportion of psychiatric patients in Mamre also say that the term 'nerves' was first given to them by doctors. For example, Ms B says: 'I had a nervous collapse. The doctor said I got a nervous collapse'. A relative, talking about Ms G, says 'Then the doctor said it was a nervous attack', and Ms G, who denies suffering from her nerves, says 'Doctor just said it was my nerves'. Ms H indicates that nerves is not her own term by describing her illness as being 'sort of attacks, you know, nervous attacks, or whatever the doctor calls it'. In the light of this finding, it is interesting that Jenkins (1988) reports that 22 per cent of her sample of Mexican-American relatives of schizophrenic patients claimed that 'they had been given the diagnosis of nerves (by medical personnel)' (p. 1239, insertion added). Jenkins interprets this finding to be attributable to 'the possibility that some relatives did not accurately remember or report physicians' findings, or that their reports were colored by their own views of the nature of the illness' (p. 1239). Another interpretation is that medical personnel in the USA may also sometimes offer the term 'nerves' to patients as a way to talk about their conditions.

Our research underscores the point that to assert a rigid distinction between folk and professional constructions of illness is inappropriate (Blumhagen, 1980). Folk models of illness are not immune to professional biomedical influence, and biomedical models are not 'purely' scientific, unaffected by social processes (Swartz, 1987a; cf. Gilbert & Mulkay, 1984). It is important to bear in mind that both folk and professional categories are not rigid and fixed.

Lessons about nerves from the Mamre Community Health Project

What interests me about nerves in the MCHP is that the term first entered the project through professionals, in their attempts to find a way of communicating with lay people. Our exploration of the term led us through many stories about nerves, like that of Elvira. Through these stories, though, we returned once again to nerves as used by professionals as a way of trying to communicate with their patients.

What does this tell us about nerves? There seems to be no question that when people from around the world – chiefly women – like Elvira suffer from their nerves, they are telling us something about how they live and how they deal with how they live. Oppression, poverty, and interpersonal conflicts can all be expressed through a range of physical and emotional symptoms, and help-seeking behaviour. This analysis does not, however, exclude other ways of looking at and thinking about nerves. Elvira's story, like those of any other person, is a complex one, and it is far too easy to try to reduce her experience to a category of 'nerves' as though this will explain her life. No category, no label can do this.

Something of the problem, or the challenge, we face in looking at nerves in different contexts is precisely in this area of reductionism. 'Nerves' is not a diagnosis in the DSM-IV sense (though it is mentioned in the DSM-IV in its discussion of culture-bound disorders). In looking for the *category* of nerves we may in our project have been looking in the wrong place. Nerves has a complex history in the interaction between health services and people. In some ways it represents an attempt to communicate between the language of the professional and the language of the lay person. In other ways, as Reynolds and Swartz (1993) show, the term may be used to block off discussion of difficult sociopolitical and interpersonal issues. Nerves teaches something about multiple and shifting meanings and interpretations, and about how people use their bodies to communicate and in attempts to improve and change their lives.

It is easy in clinical practice to reduce nerves to one category or another. Clinicians may joke about how unsophisticated people are to speak of their nerves. Others may see nerves as no more than a way of expressing political oppression. Nerves, in our experience, is not so easily categorized. It is a creation of both patients and clinicians and, if properly explored in context, opens the way for a deeper cultural and clinical understanding of people. In this respect, it is similar to many culture-bound syndromes, which will be discussed in the following section.

Culture-bound syndromes

The DSM-IV defines culture-bound syndromes in the following way:

> The term culture-bound syndrome denotes recurrent, locality-specific patterns of aberrant behavior and troubling experience that may or may not be linked to a particular DSM-IV diagnostic category. Many of these patterns are indigenously considered to be 'illnesses', or at least afflictions, and most have local names. Although presentations conforming to the major DSM-IV categories can be found throughout the world, the particular symptoms, course, and social response are very often influenced by local cultural factors. In contrast, culture-bound syndromes are generally limited to specific societies or culture areas and are localized, folk, diagnostic categories that frame coherent meanings for certain repetitive, patterned, and troubling sets of experiences and observations.
>
> There is seldom a one-to-one equivalence of any culture-bound syndrome with a DSM diagnostic entity. Aberrant behavior that might be sorted by a diagnostician using DSM-IV into several categories may be included in a single folk category, and presentations that might be considered by a diagnostician using DSM-IV as belonging to a single category may be sorted into several by an indigenous clinician. Moreover, some conditions and disorders have been conceptualized as culture-bound syndromes specific to industrialized culture (e.g., Anorexia Nervosa, Dissociative Identity Disorder) given their apparent

rarity or absence in other cultures. It should also be noted that all industrialized societies include distinctive subcultures and widely diverse immigrant groups who may present with culture-bound syndromes. (DSM-IV, 1994: 844)

From all over the world, there have been reports of behaviours which do not fit easily into Western diagnostic systems. Culture-bound syndromes which have been described include the following:

amok – violent and aggressive (even homicidal) behaviour following a period of brooding. Often this happens in a state of dissociation and the person does not recall what has happened. The expression 'running amok' comes from amok.

boufee delirante – a sudden outburst of aggressive behaviour, confusion, and motor activity. Hallucinations may also occur. It is seen typically in West Africa and Haiti.

brain fag – a response by students to schooling. Concentration, memory, and thinking problems may occur, and fatigue is reported. Somatic symptoms including headaches and blurred vision may occur. Brain fag was initially reported in West Africa. In South Africa a similar condition, isimnyama esikolweni, has been reported (Ensink & Robertson, 1996; Robertson, 1996: 217).

koro – otherwise known as genital retraction syndrome, this condition, initially reported in Malaysia, relates to such intense anxiety that the penis (in men) or the vulva and nipples (in women) will retract into the body, and that death may occur.

latah – the term is of Malaysian origin, and refers to hypersensitivity to fright, often with trancelike behaviour. There are similar conditions to be found in many parts of the world.

susto – also known as fright or soul loss, this illness is believed to be caused by the soul leaving the body after a frightening event, leading to unhappiness and sickness. It has been reported amongst Latinos in the USA, and also in Central and South America.

zar – has been reported in North Africa and the Middle East and is a form of spirit possession involving dissociative episodes which are typified by socially inappropriate behaviour. Zar may affect the person's willingness to conduct daily tasks, but is not always considered pathological. (Descriptions of syndromes excerpted from DSM-IV, 1994: 845-849, with some additions and modifications)

Nerves, or *ataques de nervios* as it is known in Latin America, is also described as a culture-bound syndrome (CBS) in the DSM-IV.

It would be possible to devote many pages – even books – to descriptions of the many CBS's described all over the world, and to questions of how to organize them into groups showing similar patterns (Simons & Hughes, 1985). The above examples were selected from the DSM-IV list because they are commonly discussed in the literature. When we examine the examples, we can see a combination of emotional, somatic, and behavioural symptoms, often with features of dissociation. What is also clear is that the codification of CBS's may depend on who is recording them. The number of reported examples of CBS's in, for example, Malaysia and Latin America may be related to the activities of mental health practitioners and anthropologists writing about those parts of the world (cf. Littlewood, 1990; Littlewood & Lipsedge, 1986). In fact, as Littlewood (1990) shows, there is at best very tentative evidence for some CBS's that have been reported. Why, then, is there so much interest in them? Acharyya (1992: 76) provides the following analysis:

> In the West, psychiatrists have tended, covertly or overtly, to play the 'colonialist game' that their own elected politicians have developed. This process has consisted of devising systems of classification of psychiatric disorders which are essentially

home-based. If such categories do not embrace migrant peoples (who do not readily fit in the classification system), these people tend to be segregated into something else. Thus they are seen as suffering from an 'exotic' condition ...

This may be an especially harsh analysis and, as we have seen in Chapter 3, there have certainly been attempts in the DSM-IV to take sensitive account of cultural factors, even though this aspect of the DSM-IV has been disappointing to many of those committed to culturally sensitive mental heath practice (Castillo, 1997; Good, 1996; Lewis-Fernández, 1996b; Lewis-Fernández & Kleinman, 1995; Mezzich et al., 1996). What is certainly true, though, is that the idea of CBS's developed when Western psychiatry was confronted with phenomena which do not easily fit what, as we have seen in Chapter 1, it has (incorrectly) regarded as its universal system of classification. Other terms for CBS's have included 'atypical' or 'exotic' psychoses (Hughes, 1996), terms which reinforce the image of Western diagnostic systems at centre stage, with other phenomena as oddities at the edges. We have seen in the previous chapter that part of the history of somatization has been the history of Western psychiatry attempting to accommodate and account for a way of being which breaks an important rule – that of physical and mental complaints being separate. A similar process occurs with CBS's, which also often break the rules of Western psychiatry. When CBS's were first discussed, the behaviour seen was often very socially disruptive, and dissociation (defined in the DSM-IV as 'a disruption in the usually integrated functions of consciousness, memory, identity, or perception of the environment'; DSM-IV, 1994: 477; see also Chapter 10) was a common feature. This strange behaviour looked to psychiatrists very much like psychosis (to be discussed in Chapters 9 and 10), but would often resolve very quickly, with sufferers commonly not having relapses or lasting behavioural changes.

As a result of this 'exotic', rule-breaking picture, a central concern in transcultural psychiatry strongly influenced by universalism has been to establish how CBS's of various types can be classified according to Western criteria. This concern is reflected in the DSM-IV definition quoted earlier. Leff (1988) explores whether CBS's can be seen as psychoses, and under what conditions.

An alternative approach, to which Leff (1988) also alludes, is less concerned with classification. This hermeneutic, or meaning-centred, approach focuses less on whether a CBS may be 'translated' into a recognizable category than on the ways in which personal and social meaning are communicated through CBS's. For example, Lee (1981), using the anthropological concepts of structure and anti-structure developed by Turner (1969), has argued that amok may be related to social pressures for control and conformity in Malaysia, and may perform an important social function in throwing these pressures into relief through the extreme nature of the behaviour. Similarly, as we have seen, nerves has been extensively analysed in terms of what it tells us about the oppression of women. In South Africa, O'Connell (1982) has suggested that spirit possession amongst rural women may be related to gender role issues in a situation in which many men are migrant workers in the cities. In addition to the communication of meaning, CBS's may, like 'nerves', affect how people interact:

> Standardised patterns of dramatic and unusual behaviour can be examined not only as instances of the shared cultural meanings they employ but as instrumental communications of distress which serve to readjust personal relationships. (Lipsedge & Littlewood, 1997: 25)

The meaning-centred approach, which can be used as a blanket term for many different specific ways of understanding CBS's in context (Hughes, 1996), implicitly goes along with a decentering of Western diagnosis as 'the truth' and, indeed, leads to an analysis of Western diagnostic systems as potentially culture-bound products in themselves. There are at least two important implications of this. First, and not surprisingly, some definitions of CBS's have focused more on meaning than on classification issues. Second, decentering Western approaches has led to an interest in Western CBS's, as has now been reflected in the DSM-IV (see definition above). I shall briefly consider each of these developments in turn.

Meaning-centred approaches to CBS's: the death of a concept?

As some theorists have shifted their interest from questions of classi-fication to questions of meaning, definitions of a CBS have also changed. Cassidy (1982) and Ritenbaugh (1982) probably go furthest along the meaning-centred path in that they offer a definition of CBS's which focuses on the meaning of the symptoms rather than on whether the symptoms occur exclusively in a particular cultural context. When Ritenbaugh (1982) speaks of obesity as a CBS, there-fore, she presents evidence that fatness and its gendered definition in the West, and especially in the USA, has led to a situation in which the syndrome of 'obesity' has come to be seen as prevalent and dangerous. There are people all over the world who are markedly heavier than average. What makes obesity a CBS of Western culture, though, is not how many obese people there may or may not be in that culture, but the *meanings* given to thinness and fatness in that particular culture.

There have been objections to this definition, chiefly on the grounds that it is so inclusive that it can be used to define *any* behaviour or condition with cultural meanings and resonance as a CBS (Prince, 1985; Prince & Tcheng-Laroche, 1987). This is, of course, true (as we shall see below). Some would argue that this is not really a problem. Hughes (1990: 140) discusses the view that reifying sets of symptoms as CBS's does not in fact guarantee these constructed entities as a sepa-rate group for psychiatric consideration. He also mentions the view that because the term CBS is used in so many different ways theoreti-cally, it may be better to drop the term altogether. In raising the ques-tion of whether CBS's are redundant as a category, Littlewood (1996: 310) points out that *all* psychiatric patterns are 'to an extent culturally constituted', and that there is also increasing recognition that 'disor-ders' are not entities 'out there' in any event, but cultural construc-tions – theories developed by psychiatrists. He argues further that there is a lack of epidemiological evidence to show without question that many CBS's exist as discrete entities. He makes the further bold assertion that 'the traditional culture-bound syndromes, which are largely the popular idea of transcultural psychiatry, are themselves likely to disappear in an increasingly homogeneous world culture' (Littlewood, 1996: 310). This strong focus on the role of Western psychiatry in constructing the notion of a CBS relates to Littlewood's insistence that there are also CBS's of Western culture, to be discussed in the next section.

Part of the problem in deciding whether CBS is a useful category at this stage is conceptual, and part of it is strategic. Conceptually, a meaning-centred approach to CBS leads ultimately to a situation in which *all* disorders can be considered as CBS's – as Littlewood (1996) mentions, culture plays a part in the construction of all mental disorder. People with a meaning-centred perspective should also have no difficulty with the concept that the diagnostic systems we use are themselves culturally constructed (Lock, 1987). If we make decisions about use of the term CBS purely on the basis of meaning, therefore, there is little argument to maintain the category. The conceptual argument against maintaining CBS as a category, however, may fail to deal fully with the probability that the vast majority of people using an instrument like the DSM-IV are interested in quick, symptom-based ways of classifying patients, and that if they are not often alerted to cultural issues they are likely to ignore them. This leads to the strategic issue.

Efforts to make the DSM-IV more culturally relevant and more truly deserving of the claim of being an internationally usable instrument have to take into account the fact that cultural concerns are not at the centre of mainstream psychiatry at present (nor have they ever been). There may be more to be gained by retaining a CBS section appended to the DSM-IV (as has in fact happened) than by a radical argument to rethink all disorders in cultural terms. This radical overhaul would be unlikely to be accepted, and would be difficult to implement practically because of the conceptual complexity of the task. Practically, though it may be misleading and problematic to have 'cultural oddities' in a separate section of the DSM-IV, this may be the most effective way of keeping the profile of cultural issues high in a discipline not especially concerned with them.

CBS's of the dominant culture

The focus within meaning-centred developments in thinking about CBS's has inevitably led to consideration of the cultural construction of the very idea of CBS's, as we have seen. Decentering from Western approaches as standard has led researchers to consider whether conditions seen commonly in the West may themselves be culture-bound. Littlewood and Lipsedge (1986, 1987) have explored the cultural meanings of overdoses with prescription drugs, shoplifting, agoraphobia, exhibitionism, and domestic sieges (Lipsedge & Littlewood, 1997), with reference to how these behaviours comment on social relationships, and can thus be understood as CBS's in the meaning-centred sense. Helman (1987) has argued that coronary-prone Type A behaviour may be understood as a Western CBS. Helman is not, of course, arguing that heart disease is confined to the West. Instead, he explores the meaning of coronary-prone behaviour in the light of Western conceptions of time and work.

Eating disorders, including obesity, and anorexia and bulimia nervosa, being so much a feature of women, have also been considered as CBS's (Ritenbaugh, 1982; Swartz, 1985a). These arguments have rested on explorations of the meaning of eating disorders in Western culture. When anorexia and bulimia nervosa are considered, however, there is also the epidemiological question of whether these symptoms are confined almost exclusively to Western contexts. There is evidence of increasing incidence of anorexia and bulimia nervosa, as well as excessive concern with weight, in minority groups in the West, and in non-Western countries (DiNicola, 1990; Lee, 1996b; Ritenbaugh et al., 1996; Swartz & Sheward, 1995). There are many possible reasons for this apparent change, not the least of which is the influence of globalization on the way people live their lives in contexts which were formerly not linked by telecommunications, the global media, the information superhighway, air travel, and massive migration (Bibeau, 1997).

Regardless of the future of CBS's of the dominant culture, and of CBS's in general as a category, it is true that disorders which either appear strange or seem to encapsulate core cultural meanings have fascinated and continue to fascinate people the world over. In the following section I shall briefly consider some of the South African debate around local CBS's.

CBS's in South Africa

When I tell people I am writing this book, many of them assume the book will be a catalogue of disorders found only amongst black South Africans. Readers who had that expectation will already have been seriously disappointed! It would, however, have been quite possible to have written a catalogue of this type (cf. Edwards et al., 1982). I hope that the discussion which follows gives an indication of why my approach has been different.

A fundamental problem with the 'catalogue' approach is that it assumes that indigenous diagnostic systems operate primarily on the same classificatory principles as the DSM-IV. As we have seen in Chapter 3, this is not necessarily a valid assumption. A recent study of CBS's amongst children and adolescents in Cape Town (Ensink & Robertson, 1996) identified five indigenous categories of distress used by indigenous healers. Only two of these, the authors conclude, were constructed empirically in a manner compatible with epidemiological investigations. In focusing on two of the most commonly discussed indigenous conditions in South Africa, I shall show how much conflict there has been in trying to understand them.

Approaches to amafufunyana

In looking at the literature on *amafufunyana*, we can see changes in the way that people have thought about the condition. According to Lund (1994), earlier studies of *amafufunyana* attempted to outline a typical list of symptoms (Laubscher, 1937; Ngubane, 1977). Ngubane, writing about illness in rural KwaZulu/Natal, describes *amafufunyana* as a form of spirit possession primarily due to sorcery. A mixture of soil and ants from a graveyard is used to make a harmful concoction which can be placed in the path of the victim. Symptoms are:

> She becomes hysterical and weeps aloud uncontrollably, throws herself on the ground, tears off her clothes, runs in a frenzy, and usually attempts to commit suicide. She reacts violently and aggressively to those who try to calm her. She is said to be possessed by a horde of spirits of different racial groups. Usually

there may be thousands of Indians or Whites, some hundreds of Sotho or Zulu spirits. (Ngubane, 1977:144)

The spirits may speak through the sufferer in a similar way to how possession and speaking in tongues is described in Pentecostal churches. For example, a Zulu-speaking woman may speak in a male voice, and in Xhosa or English. In later research, Mdleleni (1986) provides a detailed symptomatology of *amafufunyana* in three phases, in which the second phase concurs broadly with that of Ngubane, and with the work of other authors (Edwards, 1983a, 1983b; Thorpe, 1982). In later research, however, Mdleleleni (1990) interviews psychiatric patients, and finds that the term *amafufunyana* is used in different ways by different informants. In this context, *amafufunyana* emerges less as a discrete diagnostic entity with attached symptoms than as a construction or explanatory model, which patients use to make sense of their experience. It is a ready-made, socially sanctioned model, by which experiences of inner conflict can be incorporated. Its various meanings in Mdleleni's later research are analogous to the varied meanings attributed to 'nerves' by respondents in the studies of Rogers (1992) and Reynolds and Swartz (1993) discussed earlier, and has parallels with the ways the term is used in Spiro's (1991) study of serious mental disorder, to be discussed in a later chapter. Lund (1994) attempts to understand *amafufunyana* not as a set of symptoms but as a way of understanding and negotiating illness. In this respect, Lund's approach is similar to that of Littlewood and Lipsedge (1986), and Lipsedge and Littlewood (1997). *Amafufunyana*, like nerves, occurs mainly in people (often women) in relatively powerless positions. Discussing CBS's in the dominant culture in Europe and the USA, Lipsedge and Littlewood (1997: 36) describe people who are in 'a sub-dominant or marginal social position', who are, as they put it, 'extruded' or forced out of their usual prescribed social role. Under particular circumstances they may:

(i) recognise themselves extruded even further; (ii) then demonstrate what is identified as the illness in a further development of this extrusion, in a way which evokes familiar recognitions of personal distress and agency by their immediate social network by whom they are not recognised as fully responsible, which now compels others to *(iii)* reintegrate them back into their everyday social position. (Lipsedge & Littlewood, 1997: 36)

This model is an attractive one for understanding the social function of *amafufunyana*, which can occur in individuals or in outbreaks, as at a girls' high school. Ensink and Robertson (1996), however, note that descriptions of *amafufunyana* given by indigenous healers in Cape Town 'do not have the neat unitary quality of the ritualized possession states presented in the literature' (Ensink & Robertson, 1996: 159). For this reason, and because of the great variety of symptoms described in different reports of *amafufunyana*, it is possible neither to think of it as a single diagnostic entity nor as a specific set of ritualized actions with a specific set of consequences. In the case of psychiatric patients, Lund (1994) argues that *amafufunyana* provides a theory of aetiology (spirit possession) and a way of understanding what is happening, as well as a way of placing the blame for the affliction outside the patient.

The study of *amafufunyana* reflects more general tensions in the CBS's literature between trying to establish categories and typologies of disorder and trying to understand the meaning and function of disorder. *Amafufunyana* does not appear to have a single typical picture and pattern as has been suggested earlier in the literature, but it is difficult to know whether the way the term has been used has changed, or whether there was never the neat pattern suggested by earlier reports. Part of the problem here may be, as Littlewood (1990, 1996) implies, that the earlier literature on CBS's promoted the idea of there being tightly defined CBS's internationally, but the uniformity might to an extent have been imposed by those writing about them. We shall see similar issues when we discuss *ukuthwasa*.

Approaches to ukuthwasa

Whereas *amafufunyana* is viewed as a negative possession state and is commonly associated with mental disorder, *ukuthwasa* as a category is used classically to refer to a more positive state. *Ukuthwasa* is known as the state of emotional turmoil a person goes through on the path to becoming an indigenous healer. Bührmann (1982, 1983b) distinguishes between *ukuthwasa* and bewitchment, which is clearly a negative state. She argues that *ukuthwasa* arises from a positive relationship with the ancestors and is a 'calling' to become a healer. In analytic terms, *ukuthwasa* indicates an acceptance of and good relationship with unconscious material.

In the 1970s, authors were concerned to show that *ukuthwasa* was not a form of psychosis, but part of a process of becoming a healer, and essentially positive (Kruger, 1974, 1978; Schweitzer, 1977). Schweitzer (1977), for example, insisted that his informants who had undergone *ukuthwasa* were healthy people emotionally. Although *ukuthwasa* is a necessary step towards becoming a Xhosa healer, not everybody who experiences *ukuthwasa* becomes a healer, raising the question of what happens to those who do not have their social role improved through the *ukuthwasa* experience. In this vein, both Lamla (1976) and Lee (1969) point to the role that *ukuthwasa* may play in harnessing the strengths of people experiencing emotional upset. In this sense, the definition of *ukuthwasa* lies partly in the experiences of the person undergoing it and partly in the way these are handled by existing healers. Mills (1983, 1985) argues that if the outcome of *ukuthwasa* is not good, a retrospective rediagnosis of *ukuphambana* (madness) may be given. Mills (1983, 1985) argues that the term *ukuthwasa* may be used to explain a wide variety of problems and conditions, including recognized biomedical conditions such as tuberculosis. As with *amafufunyana*, it appears that the uses for the term are more broad than was once thought, an observation which is borne out by the data collected by Ensink and Robertson (1996), who found that indigenous healers in Cape Town attributed a wide range of symptoms to *ukuthwasa*. In addition to the commonly reported dreams, depressive symptoms, and anxiety, the Cape Town healers reported many antisocial features as part of *ukuthwasa*, a finding which throws into question some of the earlier views that portrayed *ukuthwasa* as almost invariably an experience with positive outcomes.

As is the case with *amafufunyana*, it is difficult to understand why there appears to be an increasingly diverse set of experiences attributed to *ukuthwasa*. Authors such as O'Connell (1980, 1982) have linked *ukuthwasa* to gender relationships in the context of migrant labour, and it is likely that as social circumstances change, so the social function of possession categories may also change. Both the terms *ukuthwasa* and *amafufunyana* do not have one single meaning. In this respect, they are similar to 'nerves', a term which, as we have seen, covers a variety of conditions and negotiations of social and personal conflict. There is no doubt that the labels have meaning but these meanings shift in different circumstances and should always be fully explored in the clinical setting. One person's *amafufunyana*, for example, may not be that of another. In Chapter 9 we will return to some of these issues as we see how different CBS labels may be used by different people to describe and understand serious mental disorder. The discussions of the current chapter, though, also raise for us questions about the relationship between social pressures and adversity and emotional states. In the following chapter, we will explore some of the ways these relationships have been thought about.

8

Culture, stress, and social upheaval

Ms Mbanga is a 35-year-old woman living with her four children and her grandson in an informal settlement near a small town. She is the sole supporter of her family. In 1976 she was in her first year of high school, but she dropped out because of the student uprisings, in which one of her closest friends was killed. She had her first child at the age of 16, in 1978, and, until her daughter was about a year old, she lived with the family of the father of the child, until he moved to Johannesburg. She has since lost contact with him. In 1979 she moved back with her parents, who were extremely angry about the birth of the child and who discouraged Ms Mbanga from spending too much time with her. Matters were made worse when Ms Mbanga gave birth to twin sons in 1980. Following extensive conflict with her family, she moved into her own shack and supported herself by selling vegetables at a stall on the main thoroughfare through the settlement.

In 1986, there was renewed political conflict in the area. Police, vigilantes, and students were amongst those involved. During the conflict (in which she had no part) Ms Mbanga was at her stall. She was shot at close range. The bullet travelled through her right arm, and she permanently lost the use of the arm. According to Ms Mbanga, she was shot by someone in police uniform. Her case was noted by a group which was monitoring 'unrest' in the area, and she was referred to a human rights legal group, which undertook to arrange a damages claim for her against the Minister of Law and Order. The lawyers engaged the services of a clinical psychologist to assist in the assessment of psychological consequences of the shooting.

The psychologist found Ms Mbanga to be living with her three children in abject poverty. Ms Mbanga was still in severe pain, and unable to work. She was also frightened of returning to her stall as her permanently disabled arm would render her more vulnerable to physical assault. It emerged in the context of the psychological assessment that Ms Mbanga had been mildly depressed since the birth of the twins. She had managed, however, to establish her small business and to ensure that her children were fed and clothed. When asked about the emotional effects of the shooting, Ms Mbanga said that her only worry was financial. She was also hoping that the shooting would help reconcile her with her parents.

The psychologist arranged for an NGO operating in the area to provide some assistance with food parcels. She wrote a detailed report for the court in which she described at some length Ms Mbanga's history and her mental state prior to the shooting. The attorney working on the case told the psychologist that a more helpful report would have shown Ms Mbanga to have been well and stress-free prior to the shooting, or at least to have demonstrated a marked deterioration in her mental state after the shooting. The psychologist felt that it would be unethical to change the report in any way. In the event, Ms Mbanga's case against the Minister did not come to anything as it could not be proved that she had been shot by a police officer.

Ms Mbanga's parents did come to her assistance after the shooting. After some time, she returned to her stall, now assisted by her mother. In 1993, she met a man who moved into her shack with her, and she gave birth to her fourth child the following year. In 1996, her eldest daughter, now 18, also had a child by Ms Mbanga's partner. She claimed he had raped her repeatedly over a period of months. When the pregnancy became apparent, the man fled and has not since been seen by the family.

Later in 1996, a newly-established NGO focusing on the emotional sequelae of violence established a satellite clinic in Ms Mbanga's area. Ms Mbanga approached the NGO for financial assistance, especially for her toddler and new grandchild. The NGO offered only psychological counselling and support groups, however. Ms Mbanga had an interview with a psychologist, who attempted to assist Ms Mbanga to talk about the trauma of the shooting ten years earlier. Ms Mbanga claimed to have forgotten all about the shooting and to be more concerned with her current financial worries. After the initial meeting with the psychologist, she decided not to return.

Stories like those of Ms Mbanga are all too common. Violence, political and domestic, deprivation, and ongoing hardship are a feature of much of the world. Large-scale migration, wars, famines, genocide, and the AIDS epidemic all have behavioural components and consequences. Whereas at one time it was thought that mental health workers should focus their interests on narrowly-defined issues of serious mental illness, there is increasing consensus that there should also be concern with ordinary people's experience of, and responses to, the pressures of living in what is often a harsh world (Desjarlais et al., 1995; Orley & Isaac, 1997; Petersen et al., 1996). How, though, do we understand Ms Mbanga and people like her? In some ways, it is obvious that someone who has suffered the way Ms Mbanga has should experience distress. From another perspective, though, and possibly from Ms Mbanga's own, it is by no means self-evident that she should experience psychological symptoms in the face of the difficulties that life throws at her. We can see from her story that twice mental health personnel crossed her path. On the first occasion, the psychologist produced a report which did not seem very useful to the attorneys attempting to gain compensation for her. On the second occasion, ten years later, Ms Mbanga herself chose not to continue to make use of psychological services made available to her.

In South Africa, in the 1980s in particular, there were many debates about the 'relevance' or otherwise of mental health services to the majority of citizens of the country (Anonymous, 1986; Berger & Lazarus, 1987; Dawes, 1985, 1986; Tau, 1989). Some arguments about 'relevance' were based on the premise that mental health professionals were rooted in a 'Western' culture, foreign to an African world-view (Bührmann, 1984; Cheetham & Griffiths, 1982; Daynes & Msengi, 1979; Hammond-Tooke, 1975; Holdstock, 1981). Increasingly, however, socio-political factors were cited as central for the apparent failure of psychology and other disciplines to address the mental health needs of all South Africans. The political violence of the 1980s and early 1990s in South Africa led many mental health practitioners to re-evaluate how they worked and should work in the future (Foster et al., 1987; Straker, 1988, 1992; Straker & the Sanctuaries Counselling Team, 1987; Swartz et al., 1990; Swartz & Levett, 1989; S. Swartz et al., 1986). Concern about, and engagement with, the psychology of oppression (Nicholas, 1993) became central. It was commonplace to claim that unless there was a nonracial democracy, mental health could not be fully realized in South Africa (Skinner & Swartz, 1989).

It seems obvious that violence and repression should have consequences for mental health:

> Wars, prolonged conflicts, and state repression lead to a flood of social and economic problems that affect well-being. The assault on communities disrupts the production of food, transportation services, and economic infrastructures; the loss of food and income leads to increased poverty and malnutrition. An additional stress on the economic base results from increased spending on arms. The violence committed against health care workers often causes a severe and lingering stress on health services. People are forced to leave their homes and communities; the dislocation breaks ties of reciprocity and sociality, increases the marginal (or illegal) status of refugees, and leads to additional trauma, the inability to mourn, and a further deterioration of standards of living. Families break up and children are orphaned or abandoned.
>
> Alongside the loss of life, the fragmentation of families, the displacement of populations, and the disruption of social and economic institutions exists a range of trauma. The problems include fear, pain, loss, grief, guilt, anxiety, hatred, sadness, and the dissolution of everyday forms of sociality, language, and experience. In turn, the breakdown in economic, social, and political systems and the weakening of a society's moral fabric often coexist with domestic, civil, and ganglike conflicts. (Desjarlais et al., 1995: 116)

Every factor mentioned above in the *World mental health* report has occurred and is currently occurring in southern Africa at present. It is difficult not to be overwhelmed by the complexity of need presented by the ubiquity of violence, repression, and their aftermath. The high rate of crime in much of the region also underscores the relationships between political and criminal violence, with many people in the region living in a state of fear or siege.

The field of research into stress and violence is enormous, and many books have been written about it. My concern in this chapter is to explore the ways questions about stress and violence are culturally elaborated, especially by professionals. Part of the problem professionals face when dealing with stress and trauma has to do with the cultural and social construction of their own social role. There is a widespread belief (some might call this a 'myth' – cf. Mossman, 1997) that mental health workers know and understand emotional trauma, and are able to heal trauma. Indeed, much that is useful has been done by mental health workers, and trauma work is an important and expanding field. My own experience, however, of working and supervising others in the trauma field leads me to conclude that the expectation of knowing what to do and how to respond to trauma can be disabling to those who want to help. This book as a whole is about thinking about culture and mental health. In the field of trauma the urgency (both perceived and actual) to do things makes thinking more difficult. It often makes thinking seem like a luxury that cannot be afforded. I hope to show here that thinking about trauma, and linking it to the ways we think about culture and mental health more generally, is not only 'affordable', but essential.

The publication of the DSM-III in 1980 was, as we have seen in Chapter 3, a major event in the history of psychiatric diagnosis. It also heralded the arrival of a new psychiatric diagnosis: posttraumatic stress disorder (PTSD). Understanding some of the history of PTSD will help us think about how we understand trauma today.

Posttraumatic stress disorder: the history of an idea

The DSM-IV diagnostic criteria for PTSD are as follows:

A The person has been exposed to a traumatic event in which both of the following were present:
1 the person experienced, witnessed, or was confronted with an event or events that involved actual or threatened death or serious injury, or a threat to the physical integrity of self or others
2 the person's response involved intense fear, helplessness, or horror. Note: In children, this may be expressed instead by disorganized or agitated behavior.

B The traumatic event is persistently reexperienced in one (or more) of the following ways:
1 recurrent and intrusive distressing recollections of the event, including images, thoughts, or perceptions. Note: In young children, repetitive play may occur in which themes or aspects of the trauma are expressed.
2 recurrent distressing dreams of the event. Note: In children, there may be frightening dreams without recognizable content.
3 acting or feeling as if the traumatic event were recurring (includes a sense of reliving the experience, illusions, hallucinations, and dissociative flashback episodes, including those that occur on awakening or when intoxicated). Note: In young children, trauma-specific reenactment may occur.
4 intense psychological distress at exposure to internal or external cues that symbolize or resemble an aspect of the traumatic event
5 physiological reactivity on exposure to internal or external cues that symbolize or resemble an aspect of the traumatic event

C Persistent avoidance of stimuli associated with the trauma and numbing of general responsiveness (not present before the trauma), as indicated by three (or more) of the following:

1 efforts to avoid thoughts, feelings, or conversations associated with the trauma
2 efforts to avoid activities, places, or people that arouse recollections of the trauma
3 inability to recall an important aspect of the trauma
4 markedly diminished interest or participation in significant activities
5 feeling of detachment or estrangement from others
6 restricted range of affect (e.g., unable to have loving feelings)
7 sense of a foreshortened future (e.g., does not expect to have a career, marriage, children, or a normal life span)

D Persistent symptoms of increased arousal (not present before the trauma), as indicated by two (or more) of the following:
1 difficulty falling or staying asleep
2 irritability or outbursts of anger
3 difficulty concentrating
4 hypervigilance
5 exaggerated startle response

E Duration of the disturbance (symptoms in Criteria B, C, and D) is more than 1 month.

F The disturbance causes clinically significant distress or impairment in social, occupational, or other important areas of functioning.

Specify if:
Acute: if duration of symptoms is less than 3 months
Chronic: if duration of symptoms is 3 months or more

Specify if:
With Delayed Onset: if onset of symptoms is at least 6 months after the stressor (DSM-IV, 1994: 427-429)

Posttraumatic stress disorder is thought to be common amongst refugees and people who have been exposed to violence. It has also been shown to put people at risk for other disorders (Breslau et al., 1997). A recent study found that of 60 children exposed to violence in Khayelitsha, Cape Town, over 20 per cent met the DSM-III-R criteria for PTSD, and 40 per cent of the children met the criteria for at least one DSM-III-R diagnosis (including PTSD) (Ensink , Roberston, Zissis et al., 1997). Almost a third of the children met the criteria for a DSM-III-R diagnosis of dysthymia, a depressive disorder in which the primary feature in children and adolescents can be either depressed mood or irritability. There was a high rate of comorbidity with PTSD – in other words, many of the children with PTSD also met the criteria for other diagnoses, notably dysthymia.

There can be no doubt that understanding how people respond to threatening situations is important for mental health workers. It is also true, however, that professionals' ideas about trauma and our responses to it are strongly influenced by social and cultural ideas, which change across different historical periods. Young (1980; 1995) has provided a detailed analysis of historical and cultural factors which have led us to place ideas about stress and PTSD at the centre of how we think about mental health challenges today. Young (1995) shows how the idea of emotional (as opposed to physical) trauma developed in the last century, and how the work of such theorists as Freud was important in the growing acceptance of the notion of trauma. The First World War affected many combatants emotionally, leading to great interest in what was then called 'shell shock'. The psychiatrist-anthropologist W. H. Rivers, whose work on 'shell shock' inspired a trilogy of highly successful novels in the 1990s (Barker, 1991, 1993, 1995), played a major part in the historical development of our thinking about trauma.

The Vietnam War was instrumental in the development of PTSD as a category, as Young (1995) shows. Part of the political impetus for establishing PTSD as a DSM-III category came from clinicians who had contact with distressed Vietnam veterans. Influential psychiatrists such as Robert Jay Lifton, well known for his work on Nazi medicine (Lifton, 1986) and on the effects of the Hiroshima bomb (Lifton, 1967), played a role in establishing PTSD. Lifton was strongly opposed to the Vietnam War, and highly critical of military psychiatry, which he saw as working centrally to return emotionally affected soldiers to the battlefield, and as acting in the interests of the military authorities rather than those of the soldier-patients (Young, 1995: 109). The establishment of PTSD as a category was a powerful way of giving voice to the view that people who had been conscripted into the Vietnam War and who were troubled on return to the USA should be seen as deserving of care and help. The diagnosis of PTSD assisted in placing responsibility for veterans' difficulties outside themselves – and in a system which made them both perpetrators of violence (in Vietnam) and victims. Young (1995) concludes his book by suggesting that as public interest in the Vietnam War changes and diminishes, interest in trauma will move to be shaped by other conflicts and issues in the world.

Constructing trauma in southern Africa

Young (1995) has shown that PTSD as a category is both a lived reality for those affected by it, and also a creation of cultural, social, and political forces. Two issues are at the centre of the creation of the PTSD category. First, there is the question of *responsibility* for trauma and for its effects. Second, there is the issue of treatment of PTSD. This second issue is, at the level of the individual patient or trauma survivor, a purely clinical question of what is most likely to help the traumatized person. At a broader level, though, the treatment issue forms part of a cultural practice which involves the use of medical language and technology to shape our understandings of social conflict. In this context, social conflict and war become *medicalized* – to be thought of in terms which use metaphors of health and illness.

The issue of responsibility was brought home to me before I had even heard of PTSD as a category. In the early 1980s, I was working in a large South African psychiatric hospital. The DSM-III was not yet in use in South Africa (it had just been published in the USA) and at that time there was far more interest in this country in British and European approaches to diagnosis. A middle-aged man was admitted to our ward suffering from severe panic attacks and intrusive dreams. It was difficult from his history to gain an understanding of why he was suffering this way. After he had been in the ward for some time, however, he revealed that he had been part of a group involved in perpetrating atrocities in the Zimbabwean War of Liberation. Although I attempted to maintain my clinical neutrality in dealing with this man, I remember feeling that somebody who had acted so viciously against civilians deserved to be in prison rather than a psychiatric hospital. Two factors increased my negative feelings towards this man. First, he had been on the side of the Rhodesian forces, and my sympathies had lain more with the liberation forces. Second, he was not a conscript, but had chosen to join the Rhodesian army. These factors taken together, I felt at the time, led him to deserve whatever emotional anguish he was now experiencing and I questioned whether, as a member of a clinical team, I would be doing the right thing to help him to deal with his very real emotional pain. As I was a trainee at the time, a senior colleague very helpfully let me out of my dilemma and took over management of the case, and I did not have to grapple with the difficulties of trying to work therapeutically with this man.

At one level, my problems with this case were all about clinical ethics. How neutral are we as clinicians? How neutral can we be? Whose interests should we be serving? Those of the individuals who happen to arrive at our doors for treatment, or those of the broader community? What happens if these interests are in conflict? All these are important questions. Clinical ethics, though, operate in a far broader social context of power relationships and issues about the ways professions deal with power issues (Swartz, 1988). The impossibility of clinical neutrality in the face of gross human rights violations by the state has been well documented in South Africa and elsewhere (Dawes, 1985; Foster et al. 1987; Straker, 1988; Swartz et al., 1990; Swartz & Levett, 1989). At another level, though, my difficulties in dealing with the patient demonstrated some of the cultural contradictions inherent in the way the mental health professions operate. From one point of view, mental health work (and health work in general) is dispassionate and value-free. Mental health practitioners are seen as scientists, operating in a context of ever-increasing knowledge to make the world better. The job of a professional is to alleviate suffering wherever it exists. My dilemma, though, demonstrated that mental health work is also about the reproduction of a particular moral order. The pain of most of the people with whom mental health practitioners deal is a relatively private matter – it occurs within families or behind closed doors. When this pain is brought into the public arena through visible trauma, though, the public role of the mental health practitioner becomes more obvious.

In the 1980s in particular, South African mental health professionals were forced by political circumstances to take up public positions with respect to issues concerning violence and state repression. 'Progressive' professionals – those who aligned themselves with the democratic forces in the country – actively researched the area of trauma, and attempted to show the damaging effects of state repression and violence (Dawes & De Villiers, 1989; Dawes et al., 1989; Straker, 1992). One issue which came up again and again in discussions of trauma and its effects at that time had to do with the idea of a single trauma being responsible for poor mental health outcomes. Violent events such as witnessing killings, political detention and disappearance, displacement, and so on, invariably occurred in communities where there had been ongoing deprivation and difficulties. Straker and the Sanctuaries Counselling Team (1987) suggested that health workers should be thinking of what they termed the 'continuous traumatic stress syndrome' rather than of PTSD, which is classically constructed as following a single traumatic experience. Similarly, Swartz and Levett (1989) record the reactions of women who had lost their homes in violence and were offered psychological support for their children in dealing with the trauma. The women, who had long lived in deprived circumstances, asked why services were being offered only now that they had no homes, and whether these services would be withdrawn once they had built their homes again. To them, the trauma of losing their homes was part of an ongoing struggle to survive, and they were rightly sceptical of what benefits could be gained from short-term trauma-focused interventions which did not take sufficient account of their ongoing context. In exploring the psychological effects of a parent's detention on the preschool child, Skinner and Swartz (1989) came to view the detention as part of a far longer pattern of difficulties faced by political activists. It was rare for detention to occur without accompanying stressors such as parents having to be on the run from authorities, separation of families, harassment, and other difficulties. Similar findings with respect to the importance of ongoing difficulties have been reported elsewhere in the world (Berry, 1995; Rousseau, 1995; Silove et al., 1997).

These observations lead us to look again at the definition of a stressor in the criteria for PTSD, and to consider where acute, severe stressors can be seen to begin and end in a violent and repressive society. As we have seen above, the first diagnostic criterion for PTSD in the DSM-IV begins:

A   The person has been exposed to a traumatic event in which both of the following were present:

1   the person experienced, witnessed, or was confronted with an event or events that involved actual or threatened death or serious injury, or a threat to the physical integrity of self or others

This is a change from the DSM-III and DSM-III-R:

A   The individual experienced 'a recognizable stressor that would evoke significant symptoms in almost anyone' (DSM-III)

A. The individual has experienced a *traumatic event* that
1   is 'outside the range of usual human experience' and
2   would be 'markedly distressing to almost anyone'. (DSM-III-R)

Clearly, across the three versions shown above, the intention is to convey a response to an unusual event which is out of the range of usual human experience and which would affect almost everyone. But what happens when we consider an ongoing political system which has been recognized internationally as criminal? How do we understand the traumatic effects of apartheid, for example? Apartheid was not an event but a system of political and economic domination which lasted for over forty years and had its roots in practices which occurred long before apartheid was official policy. Thinking about apartheid and mental health, as I shall show in the next section, can help us to outline issues we need to consider in developing an understanding of trauma, cultural changes, and their relationships to mental health.

Apartheid and mental health

This is a topic which has received considerable treatment in the literature (see, for example, Andersson & Marks, 1988; Brittain & Minty, 1988; De Beer, 1986; Dommisse, 1984a & b, 1986, 1987; Edwards, 1987; Jewkes, 1984; Lambley, 1980; Manganyi, 1973, 1991; Nicholas & Cooper, 1990; Sashidharan, 1981; Sashidharan et al., 1982; Sashidharan & Platt, 1987; Stone et al., 1979; The Lancet, 1977; Van der Spuy & Shamley, 1978; Vogelman, 1986; WHO, 1977; Zwi et al., 1988). It is easy to demonstrate that apartheid strongly affected the provision of mental health services, and that the legacy of apartheid continues to do so (Manganyi, 1991; Roth & Swartz, 1992; Swartz, 1987b, 1996). It is also true that apartheid ideology, along with colonialism more generally (Littlewood & Lipsedge, 1997; McCulloch, 1995), affected how mental health issues were understood and written about (Butchart, 1996). These effects ranged from outright racism to less obvious influences of ideology – for example, the tradition of attributing stress amongst migrant workers to cultural adjustment difficulties while ignoring the material living and working conditions of these workers (see Swartz, 1987b for a review).

More difficult to think about clearly is the question of the mental health effects of apartheid itself. Epidemiologically, though isolated studies have suggested slightly raised levels of mental illness in South Africa, there are methodological difficulties with many of them (Parry, 1996; Rumble et al., 1996). It is also very difficult to assess the impact of a global political system on mental health, and a number of authors have looked at more focused issues (e.g. Myers et al., 1982; Turton, 1986; Turton & Chalmers, 1990). Recent debates about the impact of being in a developed versus a developing country on the outcome of schizophrenia (to be discussed in the following chapter) have suggested it is important not simply to compare developed and developing countries but rather to examine the social processes affecting mentally ill people (Craig et al., 1997; Edgerton & Cohen, 1994; Hopper, 1991). Similarly, in terms of mental illness outcomes, it may be more useful to take a more focused approach, looking, for example, at the break-up of families, community destruction, forced removals, and so on.

It is a mistake to require that if a practice, like apartheid, is morally wrong, it would be necessary to 'prove' this by showing higher rates of mental illness. If such rates could not be found, then it could be argued that the practice must be morally defensible. Furthermore, to argue that people living under an oppressive system must bear the scars of that system in the form of mental illness, feels to me rather like labelling or blaming the victims. It also ignores patterns of resistance to oppression. Yet there is no doubt in my mind that apartheid did leave its mark, and continues to do so. To begin to understand this, we need to look not necessarily at rates of mental illness, but at the ways in which people interact with the world.

The Algerian psychiatrist Fanon (1970) explored the impact of colonialism on emotional development. In South Africa, similar analyses have been made by Biko (1978) and Manganyi (1973). An important role for mental health professions has been in exploring the nature of oppression and responses and resistances to it. These responses are not always, or even primarily, in the area of symptoms, but rather in the way people feel about themselves as they grow up – what they feel they can aspire to, what they deserve in life. Ways of intervening in the psychology of oppression, similarly, have to do with building constructive identities through work and social action, and not with the curing of symptoms and illnesses. This is part of the reconstruction process in South Africa, the mental health implications of which are briefly discussed below.

What is national healing?

Throughout the world, people are oppressed and violated in the name of political, religious, and philosophical ideals. Even where there is no systematic pattern of planned abuse, terrible abuses do occur, often along the fault-lines of power. Women, for example, have been violated and raped in wars for as long as histories have been recorded.

The need for national healing and reconciliation following periods of human rights abuse has long been recognized. The Nuremberg trials following the Nazi era attempted to bring to justice perpetrators, and thus to assist survivors and relatives of those who died. Chile, similarly, has been through a process of attempting to understand, and thus put behind it, its traumatic past (Becker et al., 1995). In Africa, South Africa has established a Truth and Reconciliation Commission (TRC) which, at the time of writing, is in the midst of trying to help the nation come to terms with its past.

It is beyond the scope of this book to consider in any detail the work of the TRC or to review its many and varied functions. But it is important in a book on culture and mental health with a southern African focus to think about the cultural role which our understanding of mental health and illness plays in the construction of ideas of national healing. Two of the commissioners are mental health practitioners (psychologist and registered psychiatric nurse).

A slogan of the TRC is *Truth. The Road to Reconciliation*. One of the criteria by which perpetrators of human rights abuses can apply for amnesty is if they make a full disclosure of the nature of their actions and the reasons they undertook such actions with political goals in mind. Repeatedly, in discussions of the TRC process, there are arguments that it is possible to put the past to rest only if we know what the past was – if we know what happened and why. There is a strong emphasis on the notion of the need to heal traumatic memories. For example, Hlengiwe Mkhize, a clinical psychologist and TRC commissioner, made the following statement about the TRC's work with child survivors:

As the TRC, we are strengthening our difficult memories and thinking about what young people, and children as young as six months, went through during the apartheid years ... There should be ways of establishing what happened to young people as a basis for healing and reconciliation. (Quoted in the *Cape Times*, June 12, 1997)

This model of finding the truth as a basis for healing is, of course, at the centre of psychoanalytic approaches to individual psychotherapy. It would be fair to say that most Western approaches to psychotherapy, even if they explicitly reject psychoanalytic views, depend to varying degrees on the idea that in order to solve a problem in living, one must understand how the problem came about – to get at the 'truth' of that problem. The notion of 'insight', though narrowly associated chiefly with psychoanalytic approaches, is used widely (cf. Littlewood, 1992a). How, then, does this notion of understanding the past come to be seen as a basis for collective healing? Young (1995), in discussing the history of traumatic memory, suggests:

> The pathogenic secret starts off in the nineteenth century as something located in the mind of individuals. Typically, it extends no further than the patient and the therapist. But in the 1970s, the pathogenic secret begins to enlarge, moving outward. At first, it is simply a matter of mental contagion: the secret replicates itself in the therapist's mind and in the minds of the patient's spouse and offspring. The more interesting development consists of a process in which the secret expands through mirroring rather than contagion.
>
> The psychological pathology of the individual, the microcosmos, has a mirror image in the moral pathology of the collectivity, the social macrocosmos. The collective secret is a willful ignorance of traumatic acts and a denial of post-traumatic suffering. Patients are victims twice over: victims of the original perpetrators and victims of an indifferent society. The therapeutic act of bringing the secret into full awareness is now inextricably linked to a political act. Vietnam War veterans are the first traumatic victims to demand collective recognition, and they are followed by victims of other suppressed traumas, such as childhood incest and domestic rape. (Young, 1995: 142)

In South Africa, the effects of this historical process on the creation of a category of survivors of political violence and abuse are clear. But is collective abuse the same thing as individual abuse, and are the processes the same? If we engage in national healing, are we, at the same time, necessarily healing individuals (cf. Owens, 1996)? Ramphele (1996) describes the difficult position of women whose partners died or were exiled or jailed as part of the political struggle. 'Political widowhood is a particularly ambiguous status,' she argues. 'It is both an acknowledgement and a denial of women as social and political actors in their own right' (Ramphele, 1996: 101-102). Funerals in 'struggle' South Africa were an extremely important vehicle for community mobilization and, it could be argued, for community healing. But in the large drama of the community funeral, like the even larger drama of the TRC, the needs of the individual person grieving may be sacrificed to those of the group. Ramphele describes how a political widow of the 1980s was shocked that her husband's coffin was wrapped in the flag of the South African Communist Party (SACP) when, in fact, he had been a member of the African National Congress. Ramphele comments:

> The claim that was made by the SACP stands unchallenged in history, because neither the dead man nor his widow could take back the powerful symbolic statement made by the wrapping of that flag. The claim on the dead man had a finality to it. But more importantly, it was a sign of the SACP's claim on the widow's body. This woman chose to exercise her own rights, strengthened by her intimate knowledge of her husband's political commitment, but she could have been put in a more vulnerable position if she had not had the personal resources to resist this pressure. (Ramphele, 1996: 108)

This taking over of the suffering and grief of individuals in the name of a greater communal aim is not an isolated event. I recall cases in the 1980s of individuals who had lost family members in political violence suddenly being asked to speak at meetings, and to come to symbolize something more than themselves as private mourners. This was very difficult for some of these people, but it is very hard to refuse to participate in rituals which seem to be helpful to the broader community. National healing and individual healing are not necessarily the same thing. Individuals who, through their actions or through the experience of being subjected to human rights abuses, are given the role of speaking for the nation's pain, are not necessarily 'healed', or helped by this process, and may in fact find the experience unhelpful and distressing. The sensitivity of the TRC to this issue is praiseworthy, but it is easy for us to get lost in a confusion between psychoanalytic views on how individuals can best be healed, and what is essentially the political need for a country like South Africa to find a way to meet the challenges of its future.

In Chapter 4 I raised the question of what healing systems are for and I suggested they are not only for the healing of the individual but also for social reproduction. The same can be said about all attempts to engage in national healing. In fact, national healing is perhaps centrally a communal, political effort. The role of individuals and of mental health theory in such enterprises is important, but mental health professionals need to be aware that helpful public and political processes may be unhelpful or destructive for some individuals. The PTSD history in the USA, and the political history of mental health professionals in South Africa, may give us the false hope that by using the language of individual psychopathology and healing to understand the collective, we may reach and heal more people. We need to recognize this hope for what it is – an important, and honest, desire by mental health practitioners to make as big a difference as possible to society as a whole. Collective healing, though, will never fit seamlessly with the needs of every individual. This is too much to ask. But how do we understand the interface between the individual's suffering and that of the society? We shall look at this briefly in the following section.

Social suffering

Much of this chapter has been concerned with the relationship between the individual and events and processes in the world outside the individual. As we have seen, Young (1995) has tracked the history of PTSD partly as the history of the politicization of personal pain – and of the medicalization of social conflict. A major challenge is to understand the ways that personal distress interleaves with broader social issues. There are many theories of violence, but how do we develop an understanding of violence and trauma which respects both the individual responses and constructions, and the social nature of trauma? One recent approach is to explore what has been termed social suffering:

> Social suffering results from what political, economic and institutional power does to people, and, reciprocally, from how these forms of power themselves influence responses to social problems. Included under the category of social suffering are conditions that are usually divided among separate fields: health, welfare, and legal, moral, and religious issues … [T]he trauma, pain, and disorders to which atrocity gives rise are health conditions, yet they are also political and cultural matters. Similarly, to say that poverty is the major risk factor for ill health and death is only another way of saying that health is a social indicator and indeed a social process. (Kleinman et al., 1996: xi)

The above quotation is taken from an introduction to an issue of the journal *Daedalus* devoted to understanding social suffering. What the contributors (including Ramphele, mentioned in the previous section) are trying to do is to create a way of thinking about violence and trauma in an interdisciplinary way, which does not see, for example, health problems as separate from social problems. In an article in the issue, Kleinman and Kleinman (1996) discuss how mental health problems in the context of social and political turmoil and deprivation, though shown in a World Bank report to be significant (Desjarlais et al., 1995; World Bank, 1993), are not regarded by the World Bank as the responsibility of the state. In attempting to answer the question of why the World Bank should overlook social suffering in this way, they return to some of the basic issues mentioned in the first chapter of this book. As a global institution attempting to assess the economic cost of disability, the World Bank focuses on universally recognizable indica-

tors and ignores illness experiences which vary with cultural, religious, ethnic, and gender differences. The consequences of this
universalizing approach are serious:

> Professional categories are privileged over lay categories, yet the
> experience of illness is expressed in lay terms.
>
> Furthermore, the ... [World Bank approach] ... focuses on the
> individual sufferer, denying that suffering is a social experience.
> (Kleinman & Kleinman, 1996: 14)

The authors call on us to understand suffering at the local level, and to
formulate interventions which truly serve the local needs and perceptions. They warn against accepting the ways in which the more powerful people in the world, and the media, are able to transmit their
versions of what suffering is to the world – even to sell suffering as a
marketable news item. From a complementary perspective, Farmer
(1996:280) points out that 'the poor are not only more likely to suffer,
they are also more likely to have their suffering silenced'. He also raises
the question of how we assess whether acute events, such as assault or
rape, have more negative consequences than ongoing structural violence – the violence of living for generations in poverty and under
conditions of discrimination. In this respect he echoes the concerns
raised earlier in the chapter about how we come to understand and
intervene with ongoing deprivation rather than focus only on the
obvious single traumatic event which, when people's stories are
looked at fully in context, often turns out to be more of a myth than a
reality. In the following section, we shall look at the implications of this
for how we work in response to trauma.

Towards culturally appropriate mental health responses to violence

Let us return now to the case of Ms Mbanga, discussed at the beginning of this chapter. Clearly, her contact with mental health workers

was not especially useful. Part of the reason for this, as we have seen, is that it is easier for us to think about trauma as an event rather than a process, and to try to change responses to specific circumstances rather than to make a difference to the fabric of a person's life. The material circumstances affecting Ms Mbanga are real, and psychologically important. If we do not take these into account, we cannot plan an intervention which is culturally appropriate to her.

Human rights organizations formed in response to political oppression, lawyers, and mental health workers all view suffering slightly differently. They have different professional cultures. They all have a potential role to play in assisting people like Ms Mbanga, but differences between their ways of seeing the world, if not anticipated, can lead to a wasting of professional resources. A culturally informed approach to violence requires that the different explanatory models – those held by survivors of violence, and those held by professionals and other people with different orientations, who all want to help – are recognized. When mental health work moves into the public arena in an obvious way, following a historical path similar to that mapped out by Young (1995), it is all too easy to lose sight of what mental health work can and cannot do. Healing a nation is not the same as healing an individual – and at times the two may be in conflict. Conflicts such as this make mental health work difficult, but awareness and anticipation of them may be the greatest contribution culturally informed mental health workers can make.

We need to listen to stories like those of Ms Mbanga, and to realize that our interpretations of these stories change experiences into objects and areas with which we feel we can work. This is not necessarily a problem, provided we recognize that mental health workers cannot do everything necessary in the face of violence and stress. We must recognize the limits of what we can do – this will make what we do better, as it will be neither over-ambitious nor cast in the language of groups more powerful than ourselves in the public domain. It may be tempting, for example, to talk about violence in straightforward cause-and-effect terms – terms which would help make a strong legal case for compensation. When a mental health worker speaks unselfconsciously in the terms we might anticipate a court understanding easily, however, the mental health worker has probably lost what mental health work, at its best, has to offer.

Overcoming oppression is partly a psychological process. If, however, our understanding of oppression and its consequences is truly psychological, then we must understand that human development is a long process which occurs across the history of generations. Psychological work in the field of oppression needs to consider not only what can be done about trauma now, but also how what we are doing now could potentially affect the future of communities in terms of social relationships, child-rearing, and access to resources. Crime and violence are terrible things, and mental health work is needed to help deal with them. A culturally informed understanding, though, will recognize the social embeddedness of suffering and will allow for some thought about the best ways to help. If we take context and culture seriously, we cannot provide cookbook interventions which are the same across all contexts. But we can always have with us the most important tool we have – the ability to think contextually.

9
Culture and serious mental disorder

John is a 20-year-old single man, living with his family. This is his fifth admission to a psychiatric hospital, where he has had numerous diagnoses and has been considered a complex diagnostic problem.

He grew up in a rural town close to Cape Town until the age of 10. His parents were then divorced and custody was granted to his mother. The parents agreed, however, that he should be placed in the care of his father and aunt in the Eastern Cape. Though described as an average student, he failed the second year of school. He left school at 16, after five years of education, to care for his aunt, who was dying. After leaving school he tended to his aunt's cattle and came to live with his mother in Cape Town at the age of 17, after his aunt's death. After working on a construction site for two weeks, he was first admitted to a psychiatric hospital. He had a few other jobs after absconding from the hospital, but his behaviour was described as 'inappropriate', and within six months of his first admission, he was receiving a disability grant on psychiatric grounds.

He is the second eldest of six children from his mother's second marriage. Two sisters close in age to him are unemployed; the three younger children are still at school. His half-siblings from his mother's first marriage do not live in Cape Town; six of their children (his mother's grandchildren), however, are also in the household. His mother therefore supports a household of herself, six of her children, and six grandchildren. The only other income is John's disability grant.

Mother reports that both father and mother have been *thwasa* (this is the stem of the verb *ukuthwasa* and has the same meaning) and have become healers. In addition, John's sister has received treatment for *amafufunyana* from an indigenous healer. His father's sister has been treated for mental illness (*phambana*) at another psychiatric hospital.

JOHN'S HISTORY OF ADMISSIONS TO HOSPITAL

John was first admitted at the age of 17 after exhibiting religiose and manic behaviour. On admission he was found to be in acute kidney failure and transferred to a medical unit. His physical condition was attributed to the toxicity of herbal medicine prescribed by healers of the Zionist church, who were treating him for *amafufunyana*. After a month of dialysis he was returned to the psychiatric ward, where a diagnosis of Organic Affective Syndrome was made. He absconded after five weeks and was lost to follow-up. Within a few months he was admitted to another hospital, where he was diagnosed as having Toxic Psychosis induced by cannabis (dagga). After some time on antipsychotic medication he settled and was discharged, but was again readmitted within months, diagnosed with Bipolar Affective Disorder. He was discharged a month later but within weeks was back in hospital, where again he was diagnosed with Bipolar Affective Disorder. He was placed on high doses of antipsychotic medication, but his thoughts and behaviour did not change, and he once again absconded. The present admission occurred over a year after this. Initially he settled well on antipsychotic medication but then became floridly psychotic for three weeks, then settled again. While in the ward he attempted to circumcise himself. He was admitted to a general hospital to complete the circumcision surgically.

MOTHER'S REPORT OF THE ILLNESS

The first signs of illness were noted when John returned from the Eastern Cape at the age of 17. He attended a Zionist church service where he stood up and began shouting and preaching. The next day he was excitable and continued to pray. He could not sit still and talked incessantly. Healers of the Zionist church diagnosed *amafufunyana* and prescribed herbal medicines, which did not have any effect. His sister brought him to a psychiatric hospital when he was passing dark urine, and he was treated for acute kidney failure, as noted above.

Mother was collecting herbs in Botswana for her healing practice at the time of this first admission. On her return she wanted John discharged and treated by an indigenous healer. Hospital staff tried to obstruct this by attempting to obtain a court order stating that John was to be kept in a place of safety, namely, the psychiatric hospital. This never came to pass as the hospital did not have Mother's address. She has opposed all subsequent admissions. Mother reports that the present admission occurred as John went to seek employment at the local general hospital. The social worker conducting work assessments recognized John as a former patient of the psychiatric hospital and referred him back there, and, as he was in an agitated state, he was re-admitted to the psychiatric hospital.

Mother reports that John is at present restless. He walks up and down singing hymns. He needs little sleep and irritates others with his intrusive and attention-seeking behaviour. He will say 'I love you' to any passer-by. He also claims to be receiving messages from Jesus. He hears voices instructing him to slaughter a cow to prevent people from drowning in the sea. Mother reports that these voices are those of river ancestors who are calling John to *thwasa*. The ancestors wish John to be a healer and are acting upon him through his dreams. He has also had communication from forest ancestors, who may also be involved in *thwasa*. According to Mother, it is not unusual for John to be chosen as a healer as both parents are healers, and he was born with a caul (*isingxobo*). Initially she was much opposed to the *thwasa* diagnosis for John as she did not have immediate access to the funds to pay for John's training as a healer. Now that she had accepted the diagnosis, however, she thought it essential to act quickly to avoid doing irreparable damage to John's mental state. He needed to be incorporated into the household of another healer, to receive indigenous medication and sedation to open his mind to dreams from the ancestors. These dreams would then be interpreted, and there would be ritual dancing and ceremonies with animal sacrifices. To resist this call to the ancestors would lead to *phambana*, or insanity.

One of Mother's major concerns is that John spends his disability grant without contributing to the household expenditures. When questioned, she expressed a need for support from the hospital, and for education about the illness, contact with other families with mentally ill members, and family therapy. (Adapted from Spiro, 1991)

An obvious question to ask about John is whether he should be in a psychiatric hospital at all. It could be argued from a culturally relativist perspective that he should be seen as not mentally ill but going through a culturally accepted process which is outside the framework of biomedicine. From a narrowly psychiatric perspective, on the other hand, John shows clear signs of psychosis and serious mood disturbance. His lack of compliance with treatment could be attributed to his lack of insight about his condition and, indeed, to his family's lack of insight. The fact of the matter is that he has been admitted to a psychiatric hospital no fewer than five times – it is clear that whatever systems exist outside the hospital cannot contain what is happening to him. But neither, it appears, can the hospital. He is rapidly becoming one of those patients whose folders grow fatter and fatter with each readmission as hope tends to wane regarding prognosis.

John, like very many patients in psychiatric hospitals in southern Africa, is experiencing his illness through a number of healing systems and idioms. The Zionist church has attempted to treat him for *amafufunyana*; his mother believes him to be *thwasa* and needing to respond to this call; biomedicine has dealt with serious renal problems and sees him as having a mood (affective) disorder. Drugs may also play a part in his condition. It is all too easy, when we are confronted with someone like John, to say he does not 'belong' in a Western psychiatric hospital and that he would be better off treated through indigenous healing. Ideally, this may be true, but there are many people like John who use a range of healing systems (Lund, 1994; Spiro, 1991). As we have seen earlier in this book, the idea that the world is divided neatly into a series of different cultures, each having their own particular set of healing practices, is false. In cases such as John's, which are common, such an idea may have serious effects. It could lead formal psychiatric services to claim they have no role at all to play in helping people like John.

Part of the reason John and people like him come to psychiatric hospitals is that there is no other place to go. This does not mean, though, that the institution functions just as a place of safety or custody. In the attempt to understand and, therefore, to treat people like John, staff of such institutions have to deal with their own reactions to alternative forms of treating and explaining mental disorder. They have to formulate plans of treatment which take account of these different ways of seeing the world and different resources people will use. There will often, however, be differences of opinion about how, and whether, to engage with these other resources (Swartz, 1989; 1991a). Two approaches to the issue, though different, are equally problematic. One is the view which says that biomedicine holds the only possible hope for patients and that all other approaches must be ignored or even combated. Numerous studies have shown that this is a very unrealistic way of thinking. Regardless of social background, all people in need will seek help wherever they can find it – even if this help may not seem sensible or useful to others (Boonzaier, 1985; Helman, 1994; Kleinman, 1980). A second view is that biomedicine has nothing to offer and that it is pointless to try to help. It is certainly true that biomedicine has not found any final answers to the problems of serious mental disorder, but if there were alternative services that always worked, and were always culturally appropriate and helpful, then these services would be overwhelmed with users, and biomedicine would not be used. Indeed, the wealthy from a variety of backgrounds would flock to such services (cf. Farmer, 1997).

A recent South African study (Ensink & Robertson, 1997) examined patient satisfaction with psychiatric services and African indigenous healing. The respondents in this study were Xhosa-speaking inpatients in Cape Town and their families. A majority expressed satisfaction with herbalists and faith healers, as well as with psychiatric services, but dissatisfaction with the services of diviners (amagqirha). As the authors note, there is a possibility of bias in responses as patients and families were being interviewed within a biomedical context and might not wish to say anything too negative about the services currently on offer. This possibility cannot explain, however, the discrepancy between responses regarding non-biomedical services – herbalists and faith healers versus diviners. The authors are critical of the assumption that diviners provide 'holistic' care:

> There was little evidence that diviners provided 'holistic' care; descriptions of treatment received from diviners suggest that in addition to naming the illness, prescribing medicines was the main form of treatment. In this respect the practice of diviners bears similarity to psychiatric services. Diviners frequently confirmed and thereby exacerbated bewitchment fears, without providing any further support. (Ensink & Robertson, 1997: 23)

It must again be emphasized that the authors are commenting here on reports from people currently using psychiatric services, and not on direct observations of the work of indigenous healers. Nevertheless, the romantic hope that such services will solve the problems of serious mental illness must be further called into question by such research.

The fact is that no single healing system has a 'cure' for serious mental disorder, and the responsibility of biomedicine in managing mental disorder is to do its best in the context of patients' lives. This means neither rejecting alternative approaches as a matter of principle, nor seeing other views as necessarily more 'true' than the biomedical views. We need to recognize that patients will use other services and to take them into account. Where co-operation with other services is possible, this may be a good thing, but relationships between different systems of healing are so strongly affected by issues of history and power relationships that this may not always be possible (Swartz, 1985b). A respectful relationship with other services and ways of understanding serious mental disorder, however, does not mean simply accepting that other healing services are effective. There is a tendency in the southern African literature on indigenous healing to assume that it always works and is appropriate (Swartz, 1996). This is true of no healing system, biomedical or other. Research is certainly necessary to establish the efficacy of a range of approaches to managing mental disorder, as has been suggested in Zimbabwe

(Chavunduka, 1994: 21). Just as it is incorrect to assume that all non-biomedical approaches to healing have no benefit, it is potentially dangerous to go along with a patient's faith in an alternative system if the clinician feels this system may be actively harmful to the patient. Respect for the patient and for other systems means entering into dialogue and debate, and not simply going along with what the patient or other informants may say.

The case of John (as well as the findings of Ensink & Robertson, 1997) demonstrates once again how contested the area of explanatory models of illness may be, and how there is not simply a biomedical/non-biomedical divide. The Zionist church (where John had chosen to go) had diagnosed *amafufunyana*; his mother had reluctantly diagnosed *thwasa*, and a range of labels, all of which centred on mood disturbance, were given by the hospital. We do not know the reasons for the difference in understanding between the Zionist church and John's mother. Is it simply that, like most parents, she would like her son to have a diagnosis which promises a potentially better outcome? Or is her understanding of John more accurate than that of the church? We cannot know the answer to any of the questions without more information, and in many cases there is little to be gained by trying, in a final way, to choose amongst labels given by different healers. It is more important to establish a common ground. John's mother, though working in a very different healing model from that of the hospital, expressed interest in learning more about the way the hospital sees things. One way to help patients in the context of multiple healing systems is to be aware of some of the social processes involved in the definition of serious mental disorder within the biomedical system itself, and it is to these processes that we now turn our attention.

Cultural issues in defining serious mental disorder

In earlier chapters we discussed the construction of diagnostic systems and the ways different healing systems operate. Obviously, all these principles will be brought to bear on the ways mental health workers and institutions understand and produce knowledge about people with mental disorder. These are not the only factors at play, however. Much of what we know about serious mental disorder, and psychosis in particular, comes from information gathered in the context of psychiatric institutions. As worlds in themselves, with their own sets of rules and systems of operation, psychiatric institutions have been shown to have commonalities with other total institutions, such as prisons (Goffman, 1961). Similar methods have been applied to the analysis of power in psychiatric and medical institutions and in prisons (Foucault, 1973a, 1973b, 1979). South Africa is not unique in having the history of major psychiatric institutions linked with the prison system (Butchart, 1996; S. Swartz, 1996).

I do not wish to enter here into the many arguments which exist about whether and how psychiatric institutions may act as sites of oppression – the anti-psychiatry tradition has made this point repeatedly, and there have been equally articulate arguments against this view (Ingleby, 1981, 1982; Laing & Esterson, 1964; Szasz, 1961, 1971; Wing, 1978). If, however, we are to understand the social and cultural processes involved in making decisions about serious mental illness, we need to know what transforms a person with problems into a 'case' in a psychiatric hospital (and even in talk about the person – as in the cases which have been presented in this book). Talk to and about patients, as well as writing about them in the form of notes and folders (Barrett, 1988), is only partly about finding out the 'truth' about patients – it is also about maintaining and replicating the rules of the institution. Patients who are experienced in the rules of the institution soon learn these rules and may even elicit them in interviews with staff – they learn to expect staff to behave in certain ways and to ask questions in certain ways (S. Swartz & L. Swartz, 1987). In a detailed study of the social process involved in the construction of schizophrenia in a psychiatric hospital, Barrett (1996) shows how the stories of patients are made into objects of study, segmented (as he puts it) into separate categories and then put together in terms which the psychiatric team are able to deal with. This is a necessary part of the conduct of many forms of enquiry and intervention. When, however, a patient's delusions and hallucinations are discussed under standard categories as though they were separate from the person, a process of 'repackaging' the person is taking place. Faced with a wide range of people who come to the hospital, each with a unique story, the hospital, in order to function, must impose some uniformity on patients in the form of history-taking, notes, and case discussions. This is common within other medical spheres, of course, as well as when individuals access other large institutional systems. The case notes taken by social workers, the statements of crimes taken down by police, the affidavits lawyers work with, all have uniform characteristics which make it possible for social workers, police, and lawyers to do their work. Similarly, when psychiatric hospitals or mental health practitioners talk of treating the 'whole person', what they are dealing with is a particular idea of the whole person, which the practitioners can understand and work with (Barrett, 1996; Swartz & Miller, 1992b).

In analysing the institutional construction of schizophrenia, Barrett (1996) shows how Western ideas about personhood affect this construction. He argues that a central Western conception of the person is as a whole, which organizes the parts which constitute it.

> The essence of schizophrenia becomes disintegration, where the whole can no longer exert order and control; and as a consequence the parts begin to act separately and in opposition to one another. The situation leads to a reversal of normal hierarchical relationships so individual parts can come to dominate and control the whole person. (Barrett, 1996: 294)

Barrett shows how both psychoanalytic and biological views of schizophrenia depend on this notion of an inversion of order in the person. In both approaches primitive parts of the psyche, or the brain, are seen to become dominant, with the result that 'schizophrenia is an uprising of the primitive within the civilized person' (Barrett, 1996: 294).

If schizophrenia, and by implication, other serious mental disorders, are seen as a resurgence of the primitive in an otherwise ordered person, what are the implications of this for the ways in which serious mental disorders are dealt with in institutions dealing with patients from a variety of backgrounds? The idea of mental disorder as primitive, and a resurgence of wild 'nature' in human culture is similar to many ideas about the primitive, earth-bound nature of women as opposed to men, and of black people as opposed to white people (Littlewood & Lipsedge, 1986; Swartz, 1985b). Indeed, the idea of the primitive or the savage, in women or in black people, forms some of the basis of sexism and racism. So cultural ideas and stereotypes about race and gender interact, in mental health practice, with ideas about mental illness. Staff in a psychiatric hospital in Cape Town often associated the relabelling of patients as 'cultural' as opposed to 'psychiatric' – a process I call 'cultural relabelling' – with trying to construct a story for the patient which would have a potentially better outcome (Swartz, 1991a). If, somehow, the emergence of the image of the primitive in mental disorder could be transformed into the image of the primitive of 'African culture', perhaps the person could be better helped. In much of the talk and literature produced by non-African people about mental illness amongst African people, there is the idea that there are rituals which, if only followed in 'true' cultural style by African people, will help cure serious mental illness (Swartz, 1989). In some cases, following appropriate rituals, such as those surrounding circumcision and mourning, may indeed be very helpful, but part of the hope held out for these rituals, often in the face of objections to them by African people (Swartz, 1991a), lies in trying to replace the negative primitivity of serious mental disorder with a potentially more positive primitivity. If madness can be relabelled as failure to follow old cultural ways, perhaps there can be a hope for the person in cures which lie beyond the hospital and in cultural ways which the hospital does not understand but hopes will work.

Lucas and Barrett (1995) argue that the idea of the primitive is central to much cross-cultural debate. There are, however, two images of the primitive which recur in the literature – the Barbaric perspective, which 'equates primitive society with degeneration, disruption and pathogenesis' (p. 289), and the Arcadian perspective, which 'treats primitive societies as pristine, harmonious, and therapeutic' (p. 289). Cultural relabelling within psychiatric institutions may be an attempt to replace the image of serious mental disorder as a Barbarian, degenerative process, with an Arcadian image, which implies a solution beyond the realm of biomedicine. Such relabelling may indeed be helpful, partly because the hope implicit in it may of itself have therapeutic value.

The international epidemiology of mental disorder increasingly supports the idea that rates of many serious mental conditions do not differ that markedly across cultures, and that mental health workers, however great their knowledge of and respect for other traditions of healing, will continue to be dealing with serious mental disorder (Committee to Study Female Morbidity and Mortality in Sub-Saharan Africa, 1996; Odejide et al., 1989). This view, to an extent, flies in the face of heated debates, in Britain in particular, as to whether psychotic illness may be more common amongst members of ethnic minorities, whether there may be a pattern of overdiagnosis amongst such minorities, or whether other factors, including bias on the part of researchers, may explain discrepancies observed (Fernando, 1991; Littlewood & Lipsedge, 1997; Sashidharan & Francis, 1993; Sugarman & Craufurd, 1994; Van Os et al., 1996). There has, however, been considerable discussion about whether there is a better outcome for schizophrenia in 'non-developed' societies, and it is to this debate that we shall now turn.

Does schizophrenia have a better outcome in developing societies?

The International Pilot Study on Schizophrenia (IPSS), a World Health Organization project (WHO, 1973, 1979), was designed to study schizophrenia in different cultures. It studied over a thousand patients in Colombia, Czechoslovakia (as it was at the time), Denmark, India, Nigeria, the then Soviet Union, Taiwan, the United Kingdom, and the United States. The assessment instrument used was the 9th edition of the *Present State Examination* or PSE (Wing et al., 1974). This is a standard diagnostic instrument which was translated into the languages spoken in the different centres. There were two findings which are important for this discussion – first, that it was possible to identify a core group of patients with similar schizophrenic symptoms across the world and regardless of setting and, second, that there appeared to be a better outcome for schizophrenia in the developing world. Both conclusions have been questioned by other researchers. As it is necessary to establish first what we are talking about when we speak of 'schizophrenia' before we examine the evidence about better outcome in developing countries, we will briefly first look at the universality argument and then at the more extensive debates about outcome.

Schizophrenia as a universal

As we saw in Chapter 1, there is an important approach in the cross-cultural mental health field which assumes that mental illness is universal. The IPSS demonstrated impressively that by using standard ('universal') criteria – those of the PSE – it was possible to identify a core group of schizophrenic patients in very different cultural settings but with similar symptoms. In addition to this, incidence rates for schizophrenia were reported to be comparable across centres. Kleinman (1995a) comments:

> [M]ost of the psychiatric patients who presented at the different clinical centers had to be excluded, since they did not fit the criteria. This suggested the possibility that what the study had accomplished was to use a template to stamp out a pattern of complaints that produced a more or less homogeneous sample whose similarity was an artifact of the methodology. The patients who were excluded from the study were precisely those who demonstrated the most heterogeneity. From an anthropological viewpoint, it is this very group – those who were excluded from the IPSS sample – who would be expected to demonstrate the greatest cultural difference. Second, in spite of the homogenizing template approach there were still important cross-cultural divergences. One finding was expected based on the clinical literature: certain symptoms differed in prevalence

across the centers. For example, most of the cases of catatonia were in India and Nigeria. (Kleinman, 1995a: 632)

Kleinman's argument with the IPSS is essentially that, in its quest for universals, it tends to focus on a rather limited area and to ignore or downplay important differences. In the context of many patients' being excluded from study, there are questions about how important it really is to show that a very narrowly defined set of symptoms can be shown to exist in some patients internationally. The clear and narrow definition of the sample, though, is also a strength of the IPSS approach in that it is very clear what is being referred to, and the study does not make claims beyond the confines it has set itself. In assessing the outcome data it is important to bear in mind that what is being studied is not mental disorder as a whole, but schizophrenia as defined using PSE criteria, and that large amounts of information are, of necessity, left out in a study with such a broad scope across so many sites.

The DOSMD study

The unexpected IPSS finding of a better outcome for schizophrenia in developing countries runs counter to the idea that schizophrenia is simply a biological condition which runs the same course regardless of cultural factors world-wide. A five-year follow-up of the IPSS data confirmed the picture of a better outcome in developing countries (Leff et al., 1992). There were, however, methodological problems with the IPSS. Central amongst these was the fact that the patients selected for the IPSS had all been admitted to hospital. This could be a source of bias as such facilities are more accessible in developed than in developing countries. With methodological difficulties like these taken into account, a new WHO study was designed (Jablensky et al., 1992). This study, known as the Determinants of Outcome of Severe Mental Disorders (DOSMD) study, followed up patients in Aarhus (Denmark); Agra (India); Cali (Colombia); two sites in Chandigarh (India) – one urban, one rural; Dublin (Ireland); Honolulu (USA); Ibadan (Nigeria); Moscow (USSR at the time); Nagasaki (Japan); Nottingham (United Kingdom); Prague (the then Czechoslovakia);

and Rochester (USA). Agra, Cali, Chandigarh, and Ibadan were called centres in developing countries, the remainder of the sites represent developed countries. As the authors concede, there was a bias towards urban centres, the only fully rural one being in Chandigarh. Case-finding methods were far more inclusive than those of the IPSS. Patients who participated had to be aged between 15 and 54, to have been resident in the catchment area for at least six months, and to show clearly defined evidence of psychosis or behavioural distur-bance. In addition, in the three months preceding the study, they had to have had contact, for the first time in their lives, with a 'helping agency' for the purpose of dealing with the psychotic or behavioural problems. These helping agencies varied across centres according to the resources available in the region. Patients had to have had contact with at least one of the following: psychiatric hospitals, units, or insti-tutions; psychiatric outpatient departments or centres; general practi-tioners; private psychiatrists or physicians; public health nurses or social workers; rural primary health care centres; traditional healers; religious healers; police stations or prisons; or other relevant agencies. A comprehensive assessment package was used, again with the PSE (Wing et al., 1974) as a major tool in the assessment of mental state. A total of 1 379 patients were followed up for two years. Very strict control was kept on inter-rater reliability. As it is well known that acute onset of psychosis tends to have a better outcome than does a slow, or insidious, onset, all patients were rated for type of onset of disorder. There was a dramatic difference between developing and developed centres for mode of onset: roughly half of the patients in the develop-ing countries had a very sudden onset and under a third had an insidi-ous onset in which it was not possible to demarcate clearly between the personality before the illness and the illness itself. In the developed countries, the pattern was reversed: about half the patients had an insidious onset and under a third had a very sudden onset (Jablensky et al., 1992: 25).

Numerous methods were used to assess outcome over two years. Table 9.1 is adapted from the WHO report.

Table 9.1 Percentage of patients in developing and developed countries falling into selected categories of course and outcome variables

Course and outcome category	Developing countries	Developed countries
1 Remitting course with full remission	62.7	36.8
Continuous, or episodic psychotic illness without full remission	35.7	60.9
2 In psychotic episodes 1–5 % of follow-up period	18.4	18.7
In psychotic episodes 76–100 % of follow-up period	. 15.1	20.2
3 In complete remission 0 % of follow-up period	24.1	57.2
In complete remission 76–100 % of follow-up period	38.3	22.3
4 No antipsychotic medication throughout follow-up period	5.9	2.5
On antipsychotic medication 76–100 % of follow-up period	15.9	60.8
5 Never hospitalized	55.5	8.1
Hospitalized for 76–100 % of follow-up period	0.3	2.3
6 Impaired social functioning throughout follow-up period	15.7	41.6
Unimpaired social functioning for 76–100 % of follow-up period	42.9	31.6

(Adapted from: Determinants of Outcome of Severe Mental Disorders – DOSMD – Jablensky et al., 1992: 64)

As the table shows, on all but one of the six criteria used to measure outcome, substantially greater proportions of patients in developing countries showed good outcome than did those in developed countries. Some of the criterion measures are, of course, affected by availability of services – one might, for example, expect more hospital admissions and use of antipsychotic medication in countries where there are more hospital services available and antipsychotic medication is easier to obtain and afford. Not all the outcome measures, however, depend on such factors and the magnitude of some of the differences is large – for example, patients in developed countries are 2.6 times as likely to have social impairment throughout the follow-up period than are their counterparts in developing countries.

The authors considered the possibility that the better outcome in the developing countries was due to the more acute presentations in developing countries. Acute onset, it will be recalled, tends to have a better outcome than insidious onset, regardless of where the patient is situated. They therefore reanalysed the data taking this into account. While the dramatic picture of Table 9.1 was indeed moderated when mode of onset was taken into account, the differing pattern of course, with developing countries showing a better outcome, was maintained. The authors also considered the possibility that there might have been a greater frequency of atypical brief psychoses in the developing country sample but conclude there is insufficient evidence to support this view (the question of brief psychosis will be considered in the following chapter). They conceded that there may be different conditions which present with identical symptoms. If this were the case, there could be two conditions, identical in terms of symptoms, but with different causes and genetic patterns, one of which could have a better outcome than the other. The better outcome condition could be more common in developing countries. At present, the authors note, it is not possible to test this hypothesis as we do not have 'established genetic markers, indicators of aetiology or other underlying mechanisms of disease' (Jablensky et al., 1992).

Having extensively considered a range of possible alternative explanations for their findings, the authors concluded they had found a real difference in outcome, a difference which for them confirms the earlier findings of the IPSS. What, though, explains this difference?

> [A] strong case can be made for a real pervasive influence of a powerful factor which can be referred to as 'culture'. Unfortunately, neither the IPSS nor the Outcome study could penetrate in sufficient depth below the surface on which the impact of this unknown factor was established – tentatively in the IPSS and definitively in the present study. (Jablensky et al., 1992: 88-89)

What is inside what Edgerton and Cohen (1994: 230) have termed this 'black box' of culture? Jablensky et al. (1992) do not claim to know the answer, and they admit they are applying the broad label of culture to describe differences in life in the different settings, which they have not sufficiently studied. One possible contributory factor, they argue, though not one which can explain all the differences, is that of Expressed Emotion, which I shall now briefly discuss.

Studies in London demonstrated that patients with schizophrenia were more likely to relapse if their relatives were highly critical of them or emotionally over-involved with them (Brown et al., 1972; Vaughn & Leff, 1976). Leff and Vaughn (1985) operationalized this observation into a measure of families' involvement with patients with schizo-phrenia, the measure being known as Expressed Emotion (EE). A series of studies in India (Leff et al., 1987, 1990; Wig, Menon, Bedi, et al., 1987; Wig, Menon, Leff, et al., 1987) demonstrated not only that the proportion of households with at least one high EE relative was lower in India than in the West, but also that the association between low EE and better outcome for schizophrenia was maintained in different settings. EE has been studied in many parts of the world (Barrelet et al., 1990; Karno et al., 1987; Kuipers & Bebbington, 1988, Vaughn et al., 1984; see also Leff, 1988, for a review, and Kaslow et al., 1995, for a review of cultural issues in family theory), and evidence has been provided in support of the view that more tolerant family atti-tudes towards persons with schizophrenia and other disorders may be associated with better outcome. There is also ample evidence that intervention with families of patients with schizophrenia (in part designed to give information and hence to assist family members to be more tolerant) has a beneficial outcome (De Jesus Mari & Streiner, 1994; Kuipers, 1996; Penn & Mueser, 1996). If such attitudes are prevalent in developing countries, then this may explain a better outcome for schizophrenia. Similarly, it has been argued, if there is an extended family to share the burden of mental illness, then it should follow that there will be more tolerance, lower EE, and hence better outcome. None of these issues has been conclusively proven, and there is considerable debate about this type of argument, as we shall see in the following section. Jenkins (1991) has provided a detailed critique of the EE concept based on her work with Mexican-Americans with schizophrenia (Jenkins, 1988). Some of the issues she raises will be taken up in the following section; at this point it is important simply to note her view that EE cannot be considered as an entity separate from differing conceptions of illness itself. If we follow this line of reasoning, EE may be affected by the extent to which relatives believe the illness to be of chronic course and likely to have good outcome. This argument returns us to thinking about the role of explanatory models in affecting the course of disorder.

In summary, the DOSMD study (Jablensky et al., 1992) appears to have provided strong evidence for a better outcome for schizophrenia in the developing world, but apart from suggesting EE as one factor which may explain differences, it does not purport to understand the differences it has observed and has attributed to 'culture'. Indeed, the authors lay down an important challenge to researchers and clinicians interested in the effects of culture on the course of serious mental disorder:

> The contribution of the present study ... is not in providing the answer but in clearly demonstrating the existence of the question. (Jablensky et al., 1992: 89)

In the following section we shall briefly note other studies with similar findings to that of the IPSS and the DOSMD, and we shall then consider some of the emerging debates in the area.

Other studies and comments on the IPSS and DOSMD approach

An early follow-up study of mental disorder in Cape Town amongst coloured people, though methodologically at an earlier stage of development than the IPSS and DOSMD studies, provides some evidence to suggest that outcome was better for psychosis (if not for other disorders) in Cape Town than in centres in the developed world (Gillis & Stone, 1973). In Mauritius, Murphy and Raman (1971) demonstrated a better outcome for schizophrenia than in Britain, though there may be some difficulties with their case definition – favouring 'mild' cases (Cohen, 1992: 54), or even cases which in Britain would not qualify for a diagnosis of schizophrenia (Leff, 1988: 154). Waxler (1977, 1979) reported a better outcome for schizophrenia in Sri Lanka, attributing her findings partly to a large and robust Sinhalese family, and to her finding that Sinhalese people are likely to attribute mental illness to supernatural causes, and hence are less likely to stigmatize the mentally ill. Leff (1988: 151-162) reviews a number of studies, including those cited here, not all of which find a better outcome for schizophrenia in the developing world but which, taken as a whole, suggest the trend for a better outcome indeed exists.

In similar vein, Warner (1985, 1994) attributes better recovery from schizophrenia in the Third World in part to greater participation in the economy by disabled people. High unemployment rates would make it more difficult for people who have suffered from a mental disorder to find work and, hence, to play a meaningful role in society, which would lead to better reintegration. In a subsistence economy, furthermore, Warner argues, 'people with mental illness may perform any of those available tasks that match their level of functioning at a given time' (Warner, 1994: 157). In the context of such an economy, where there are always jobs to do, 'unemployment' becomes a meaningless term, and the damaging effects of unemployment are avoided. In Warner's opinion:

> The general conclusion is unavoidable: schizophrenia in the Third World has a course and prognosis quite unlike the condition as we recognize it in the West. The progressive deterioration

which Kraepelin [who first described schizophrenia, or *dementia praecox*, as he called it] considered central to his definition of the disease is a rare event in non-industrial societies, except perhaps under the dehumanizing restrictions of a traditional asylum. The majority of Third World schizophrenic people achieve a favour-able outcome. The more urbanized and industrialized the setting, the more malignant becomes the illness. (Warner, 1994: 157; insertion added)

Before the publication of the final DOSMD report reviewed above (Jablensky et al., 1992), but after the publication of a preliminary report (Sartorius et al., 1986), Cohen (1992) suggested, in the face of the evidence from a range of studies, that the case for there being a better outcome for schizophrenia in the Third World has yet to be proven. Some of Cohen's arguments were refuted, disputed, or modi-fied by commentators on his article, all of them key researchers in the field (Hopper, 1992; Sartorius, 1992; Warner, 1992; Waxler-Morrison, 1992), and it is not my intention here to go into all the intricacies of the debate. An article by Edgerton and Cohen (1994) subsequent to the final DOSMD report, with a response from the DOSMD team (Jablensky et al., 1994), takes the debate further. What is important and useful about the debate is that it makes clear some central ques-tions not only for cross-cultural research into schizophrenia, but for cultural research in the health and social service field more generally. Some of these are reviewed below.

1 The need for more ethnographic information

A central point made by Cohen (1992) is that even if data have been presented suggesting a better outcome for schizophrenia in the Third World, the mechanism for this difference has yet to be demonstrated. Discussing the work of Waxler, he says:

Although Waxler may offer Sinhalese culture as the reason schizophrenia seems to follow a relatively benign course in Sri Lanka, she never provides us with ethnographic evidence to support these claims. (Cohen, 1992: 60)

In concluding his article, he argues further:

> [W]e need to conduct ethnographic research into the lives of individuals with schizophrenia. We cannot merely employ follow-up strategies, we need to *follow* patients ... Long-term, ethnographic information about persons with schizophrenia is required to assess the current debates in cross-cultural psychiatry ... Until more research is moved out of the clinics and hospitals and into the day-to-day lives of schizophrenics, our impressions of this mental disorder will remain incomplete and inaccurate. (Cohen, 1992: 70, his emphasis)

As has been quoted earlier in this chapter, the authors of the DOSMD report agree that further research is needed into the variable of 'culture', which they do not define. One way of doing this is through the detailed hermeneutic research of the type Cohen (1992) is suggesting. Waxler-Morrison (1992), as Waxler was known by 1992, agrees with Cohen (1992) that more ethnographic research on schizophrenia is needed, as does Sartorius (1992), representing a WHO view. Waxler-Morrison refers to the important work of Estroff (1981), who studied psychiatric patients in a community in the USA. So determined was Estroff to understand the experience of such patients, that she even took psychotropic medication herself for a time so that she would gain an experience of the side-effects. As Hopper (1992: 95) puts it, much of the hypothesizing we do about an outcome for schizophrenia in the Third World 'goes on in a virtual ethnographic vacuum'. Warner's (1994) highly sophisticated statistical analyses, for example, are presented in a context which makes broad generalizations about formal and informal economic activity in many parts of the world. Clearly, the more detail we can have on the everyday lives of people with mental disorder around the world, both inside and outside of institutional care, the better.

2 The need for theoretical development

This issue relates very strongly to the first. Cohen argues that we need to understand the meaning of all measures used in studies for the respondents themselves. If we do not do this we cannot be sure what we are measuring. This involves more than accurate translation and back-translation – it requires us to find out, as far as we are able, whether the meaning we give to any instrument has the same meaning for our respondents. This meaning will depend on the social context and beliefs of respondents. In Chapter 5 we saw how Obeyesekere (1985) has argued that some of the hopelessness which, in the West, is part of the negative syndrome of depression, may be a desired state of consciousness for Buddhists in Sri Lanka. Similar cultural factors may affect any assessments in studies such as the IPSS and the DOSMD, as well as other studies.

In asking us to open the 'black box' (Edgerton & Cohen, 1994) of culture, Cohen (1992) is asking not just for more information, though this is central. He is also propagating a relativist position which says that it is essential not to impose our own assumptions on data, and on the ways we ask questions. This has implications for the data-collection process, and recalls the debates between different methodologies which we discussed at the beginning of this book. Interestingly, in trying to develop our theoretical understanding of Expressed Emotion, Jenkins and Karno (1992) also attempt to open up a 'black box' concept. These authors are asking us to make explicit the way in which researchers' own cultural assumptions about the world affect the design of their studies and the ways they ask questions about the world. These assumptions relate to the next central issue.

3   The problem of dualism and the politics of labelling

Edgerton and Cohen (1994) discuss the five centres used by the DOSMD to represent the 'developing world'. As we have seen, these centres are Agra (India); Cali (Colombia); two sites in Chandigarh (India) – one urban, one rural; and Ibadan (Nigeria). They argue:

> [O]ne thing is obvious. These five centres do not begin to represent the full range of social or cultural diversity in what might be called the developing world, nor can they be said to be typical of that world ... (Further, that the three north India sites should be

treated as independent cases is questionable from a statistical viewpoint because they are culturally so related.) It is difficult to comprehend how findings about differences between 'developing' and 'developed' societies could be considered 'conclusive' when they are based on this sample. (Edgerton & Cohen, 1994: 225)

As we have seen in Chapter 3, there are many stereotypes about the differences between 'traditional' and 'modern' people, about the 'Western' and the 'non-Western' ways of life, and so on. Does the assumption that the world can be neatly divided into 'developed' and 'developing' sectors play a part in how we have come to know about outcome for schizophrenia? On this issue, I find Edgerton and Cohen's (1994) argument especially persuasive. Five centres, four of them urban, and three from the same country, do not represent 'the developing world'. Similarly, the countries representing the 'developed' world cannot be seen necessarily to represent accurately the range of 'the developed world'. Edgerton and Cohen (1994) make the further point that underlying the DOSMD study is the assumption that within any given centre – Ibadan, say – the patients are culturally from the same group. This is almost certainly not the case, especially in modern cities in the context of world-wide mobility and urbanization (Harpham & Blue, 1995). Writing from Zimbabwe, Patel and Winston (1994) call for regional as opposed to multinational studies, arguing that regional studies are far more likely to avoid what they term the 'premature construction of standard forms of diagnosis and classification' (Patel & Winston, 1994: 439). Stereotyping of mental illness in developing countries is likely to decrease with regional studies, they argue further, and studies are more likely to relate in a practical way to the mental health resources (biomedical and non-biomedical) in those countries. It is almost inevitable that large-scale international studies will lead to glossing over of detail, and to the false assumption that people are culturally all the same just because they live in the same geographical area, or are given the same label. This type of assumption has political underpinnings well demonstrated in the South African context.

South African scholarship in the social sciences in the 1980s has helped us see how attractive dualism is in our thinking – in separating the 'traditional' from the 'modern', the 'Third World' from the 'First World', and so on (Boonzaier & Sharp, 1988). These dualistic assumptions, especially those about 'culture' and ethnicity, it has been shown, helped create academic knowledge which fitted neatly with apartheid ideology – an ideology which depended for its very existence on dualism – between white and black people (Boonzaier & Sharp, 1988; Sharp, 1980). Bearing in mind the argument that the notion of a neatly divided world is socially constructed (Sharp, 1988), could it be that more ethnographically-informed research in various settings might reveal not only more cultural information about people with schizophrenia in different parts of the world, but also something of the cultural diversity which may exist in the developing countries? Some of this information may well be of relevance to how schizophrenia is managed and progresses.

Part of the argument of contributors to the Boonzaier and Sharp (1988) volume, as we have seen, is that theoretical dualism within the social sciences meshed well with apartheid ideology. In the area of South African research into the outcome of serious mental disorder, this social climate has had some effect. Gillis and his colleagues (Gillis, 1986b, 1987; Gillis et al., 1986a, 1986b, 1989; Gillis, Jakoet, et al., 1987; Gillis, Trollip, et al., 1987) studied outcome of schizophrenia amongst white, coloured, and African patients in Cape Town, using a careful methodology heavily influenced by the IPSS. Interestingly, outcome at two years was not substantially different between whites and Africans (Gillis, Jakoet, et al., 1987), though Africans showed higher rates of disturbed behaviour, and whites more severe symptoms. Unfortunately, in contrast with the careful epidemiological methods applied, there is less emphasis on going beyond given categories ('white', 'coloured', 'African') to explore what, if anything, these labels might mean. In examining compliance with medication amongst African patients, Gillis et al. (1989) argue that African patients subscribe to

the traditional African view that the causation of mental illness lies in a disturbance in the whole being and takes account of powers in the unseen world including the protection of the ancestors, witch-craft and spirit forces. The psychiatrist's pills are not enough. The traditional healer, on the other hand, operates within the patient's own milieu, his remedies being non-medical in the form of rituals, social acts and animal sacrifices. (Gillis et al., 1989: 207)

This argument is put forward in the absence of the patients themselves having been asked about their beliefs, so they represent an *assumption* by the authors about the beliefs of patients. Cultural difference is read into the fact that the patients are Africans, rather than discovered from finding out about this from them. Gillis et al. are able to show the very useful finding that a home visit helps to make patients substantially more compliant with medication; their analysis of the reasons for non-compliance, however, relies on dualistic assumptions. These assumptions, though perhaps more obvious in the context of South African psychiatry during the apartheid era, are seen in a very similar way in major international psychiatric research.

A recent article which has bearing on the question of the developed/developing world duality has recently been published by Craig et al. (1997). These authors have re-analysed the DOSMD data and have found that the course of schizophrenia is indeed best predicted by the centre in which patients lived. They found, however, that two of the centres in the 'developed' group, Prague and Nottingham, fitted best in their outcome pattern with 'developing' country centres, excluding Cali. This is an exciting finding, first because it begins to break down previous simple dualism, and it is a step towards opening the

'black box' of imputed cultural effects on outcome – in particular of stigma, family support, availability of treatment and rehabilitation services, social relationships, and available employment for disabled individuals. (Craig et al., 1997: 232)

When we know more of what we are talking about behind the labels of cultural difference and the developed/developing divide, then we will have more accurate information of use to people with schizophrenia and those wishing to help to them.

4   The diagnostic question – is this schizophrenia?

The DOSMD, as we have seen, was scrupulously careful about defining its diagnostic terms, but leaves open the question of whether there could be more than one condition with identical symptomatology. Warner speculates that Third World samples may include

> more cases of, say, malarial psychosis, nutritional disorders or drug-induced psychoses which would tend to have a better outcome than schizophrenia. (Warner, 1992: 87)

In raising this possibility, Warner is referring to a large literature which suggests that brief psychoses 'clinically indistinguishable from schizophrenia' (Warner, 1994: 170) may well be a feature of mental disorder in the Third World, for various reasons. This possibility will be considered in the following chapter.

Concluding comments

It is not possible in the space of this book to give full justice to all the issues about serious mental disorder and culture. In this chapter I have focused on two key issues: cultural factors in defining serious mental disorder, and the debates concerning schizophrenia, in particular, and its outcome in the developing world. There is much evidence to support the 'better outcome' hypothesis, but important methodological and theoretical questions have been raised, and re-analysis of DOSMD data raises further questions. Part of the reason the work looking at outcome for schizophrenia is so important lies not in the question of whether there is or is not a better outcome in developing countries. Instead, thinking about the issue helps us clarify what are important general questions for our field. In the following chapter, dealing with what I term the 'borderlands' of the field, the echoes of these important questions will be heard again and again.

10

Thinking at the borderland

I recently met a European colleague who was visiting South Africa, and I was discussing with her plans others and I are making for a project to assist parents and infants in an informal settlement near Cape Town. She suggested that instead of working with people in an informal settlement, it would be more culturally sensitive to begin working with people in a remote rural area. This would allow us to understand African culture without the harmful effects of urbanization and living in an informal settlement. Once we had understood this rural culture we could begin to understand the changes wrought upon it by urban life.

In one sense my colleague was right. There would be much to be gained from understanding rural child-rearing practices, and from contributing to the excellent knowledge already available about such practices in Africa (see, for example, Ainsworth, 1967; LeVine et al., 1994). In another sense, though, she was privileging the experience of the rural African, and saying that it was more 'real' or 'truly cultural' than urban experience. In the context of a 'creolizing world' (Bibeau, 1997), the search for the true rural village, homogeneous and untouched by other cultures, becomes more and more attractive but, in fact, may be more and more illusory. What village in South Africa, for example, however remote, has not been affected by apartheid, migrant labour, and conflict? Why, furthermore, should we be searching for the true rural roots of African people, as a matter of principle, when we are far less likely to do so for other people (Swartz, 1985b)? Answers to questions about true rural African practices are partly empirical, but also represent a view of the world neatly divided into different 'cultures'. In this neatly-divided world, the image of which people of different academic and political persuasions have a stake in maintaining (Swartz, 1996), there are also neat categorizable illnesses which fit a standard diagnostic system. Those illnesses which do not fit that system can be understood in terms of another, local system which is complementary to the standard one.

As we have seen throughout this book, the idea of neat classifications of people, disorders, healing systems, and so on, does not hold up in the face of a far more complex interplay of different ways of seeing and being in the world. In this chapter, the last in this book to deal directly with clinical symptoms as such, we shall discuss a range of issues which present challenges to the image of the neatly-divided modern world of psychiatry. As we shall see, some of these issues come from cross-cultural challenges within mental health care, and others are more clearly associated with cultural changes in the dominant 'Western' world. First, I will look at debates concerning transient psychosis, and what these may imply for how we view the world. Second, I will examine the field of drugs, alcohol, and psychotropic medication and consider how this field also forces us to rethink our standard ideas about mental health and illness. Finally, I will consider current interest in dissociation, and the implications this holds for our field.

The question of transient psychosis

As we saw in the previous chapter, the strong evidence for a better outcome for schizophrenia in developing countries has led some to suggest that transient psychoses may be a feature of the developing world (Warner, 1994). The DSM-IV makes allowance for the diagnosis of brief psychotic disorder with the following diagnostic features:

> The essential feature of Brief Psychotic Disorder is a disturbance that involves the sudden onset of at least one of the following positive psychotic symptoms: delusions, hallucinations, dis-

organized speech (e.g., frequent derailment or incoherence), or grossly disorganized or catatonic behavior (Criterion A). An episode of the disturbance lasts at least 1 day but less than 1 month, and the individual eventually has a full return to the premorbid level of functioning (Criterion B). The disturbance is not better accounted for by a Mood Disorder With Psychotic Features, by Schizoaffective Disorder, or by Schizophrenia and is not due to the direct physiological effects of a substance (e.g., a hallucinogen) or a general medical condition (e.g., subdural hematoma) (Criterion C). (DSM-IV, 1994: 302)

The DSM-IV states that such disorders are thought to be rare and may follow traumatic experiences (as in PTSD). Under 'specific culture features' the DSM-IV notes:

> It is important to distinguish symptoms of Brief Psychotic Disorder from culturally sanctioned response patterns. For example, in some religious ceremonies, an individual may report hearing voices, but these do not generally persist and are not perceived as abnormal by most members of the person's community. (DSM-IV, 1994: 303)

There is no statement in the DSM-IV that brief psychotic disorders are more likely to be common in the developing world, an omission which runs counter to the views of Warner (1994) and those of many other authors. In my own research with psychiatrists in training in Cape Town, I found a widespread belief in a florid, rapidly resolving psychosis amongst African patients (Swartz, 1989). Some authors have sought to differentiate 'true' psychosis from possession states such as *amafufunyana* and *ukuthwasa* (Bührmann, 1977, 1982; Kruger, 1978), which may possibly link with the distinction the DSM-IV makes with 'culturally sanctioned response patterns', as quoted above. But is there something more to the apparent preponderance of brief psychotic states in the developing world?

There has long been controversy about the existence of acute remitting psychoses (Menuck et al., 1989). Susser & Wanderling (1994), however, found that what they termed 'nonaffective acute remitting psychosis' (NARP) was roughly ten times as common in terms of incidence in developing as opposed to developed countries, with women outnumbering men approximately two to one in all settings. Using data in Chandigarh, India, Susser et al. (1995) provide evidence to suggest that acute transient psychoses did not have a significant mood or affective component, as has previously been argued, and were easily distinguishable from schizophrenia in terms of duration of disorder. Susser et al. (1996) suggest a DSM-V diagnosis of NARP, with four central criteria: 1) nonaffective; 2) acute onset (over less than two weeks); 3) recovery within a brief duration (less than six months); and 4) psychosis broadly defined. They point out that since the 1950s psychiatrists in developing countries have reported treating large numbers of acute onset, florid psychoses of variable clinical features, which resolve rapidly with or without treatment (Susser et al., 1996). One of the names given to these psychoses has been 'atypical' psychosis because the clinical picture does not fit the standard picture, but these psychoses are in fact common in many parts of the world. Other terms used have been 'brief reactive psychosis, hysterical psychosis, bouffe delirante, cycloid psychosis, schizophreniform disorder' (Collins et al., 1996: 178).

It has been shown repeatedly that physical conditions including infections by parasites or other means may lead to reversible psychotic states – malaria is a particular problem in Africa (Asuni et al., 1994; Desjarlais et al., 1995; Leff, 1988). Collins et al. (1996) re-analysed IPSS data from Ibadan, Nigeria, and Agra and rural Chandigarh, India. They found an association between fever and acute brief psychosis in all three sites, evidence which tends to support the idea that brief psychoses may be of infective or similar organic origin. They found further, however, an association between brief reactive psychosis and departure from or return to the parental village among women across all three sites. For men, job distress was associated with acute brief psychosis in Ibadan and Agra. These findings suggest that both biological and psychosocial factors may play a role in the development and presentation of brief reactive psychoses.

Separating out biological and psychosocial factors in psychiatric symptoms may not be easy, and a substantial overlap between physical and psychiatric morbidity has been shown in general practice settings (Kisely & Goldberg, 1996). Just as we may, however, be over-hasty to attribute physical symptoms amongst distressed people to somatization (see Chapter 6), there may be a danger in attributing psychoses purely to biological causes. Leff (1988: 168) refers to Asuni's (1967) analysis of malarial psychosis. According to Asuni, there are three possibilities to explain schizophrenic symptoms in the presence of parasites. First, the parasites may affect the brain, causing organic psychosis. Second, a stress-induced psychotic episode may occur when the patient becomes aware of having contracted malaria. Finally, the patient may, by chance, contract both conditions simultaneously, but there may not be a relationship between the psychosis and the malaria. It would be expected that where malaria is common, it would generally occur amongst people with psychotic disorders. Only in the first case can the malaria be said to be 'causing' the psychosis.

Simply to speculate about organic factors and their co-occurrence with psychosis, therefore, may not be enough. Some presentations of psychosis which are thought to be more common in the Third World – notably, catatonic and highly excitable states – have been shown to also occur amongst people with known fever or other organic illness. There is also, as we have seen, emerging evidence that it may be possible to distinguish brief psychoses from other psychoses on psychosocial grounds. Trying to separate biological from psychosocial causes may be especially useful in planning treatment and prevention strategies, but the time may be ripe for us to abandon the question of whether a psychotic episode is either biological or psychosocial. Biological psychiatry has made great strides in demonstrating the biological components of what was formerly considered 'functional' illness – or illness of non-organic origin, and developments in the social sciences have shown us how important sociocultural and psychological factors are in the aetiology and prognosis of organic illness (Eisenberg, 1995). The apparent preponderance of brief psychoses in the developing world may well help us begin to understand the intertwining of organic and social factors more clearly. This 'borderland' area of mental illness is crucial in providing information about possibly the central preoccupation of Western psychiatry at present – the status and implications of biological psychiatry. Perhaps ironically, it can now be argued that an understanding of sociocultural factors may help us develop more focused hypotheses about biological factors. Discussing acute psychoses, Collins et al. (1996) write:

> Investigating these disorders in the developing world, where they occur more frequently, and pursuing leads along sociocultural and gender lines, can reveal important facts about the biology as well. (Collins et al., 1996: 191)

Alcohol, drugs, and culture

Selected epidemiological information on alcohol and drugs

There is an enormous amount of information internationally on the epidemiology of alcohol and drugs (including tobacco). For the purposes of this discussion, only a few key features will be highlighted.

Alcohol

The 1993 World Development Report estimates that alcohol-related diseases affect 5 to 10 per cent of the world's population annually (Desjarlais et al., 1995: 87). Health costs of alcohol affect not only the drinkers themselves, but also others around them, including unborn children, who may develop foetal alcohol syndrome (Zuckerman & Brown, 1993). There have been major expansions of the liquor industry, and in consumption of alcohol in low-income countries (Desjarlais et al., 1995: 91). In Nigeria, 'the manufacturing sector to which the breweries belong, recorded an annual average growth of 15 per cent between 1970 and 1984' (Peltzer, 1995: 43), and in Papua New Guinea, beer consumption doubled every four or five years during 1962-1980 (Desjarlais et al., 1995: 95). A similar picture of increase has been shown in South Africa (Parry & Bennetts, in press). The health burden of alcohol may be greater in lower-income countries; for example, the death rate from cirrhosis of the liver (a condition associated with alcohol abuse) in Mexico and Chile is over four times that of the USA (Desjarlais et al., 1995: 95). Alcohol is also associated with violence and road traffic accidents. As Orford (1991) notes, the old stereotype of the 'alcoholic' as a middle-aged man has broken down with increasing awareness that alcohol is used amongst all age groups including the elderly and teenagers, and with evidence of increases in drinking amongst women – younger women in particular (Doyal, 1995). Ben-Tovim (1987: 108-109) found that a substantial percentage of referrals for psychiatric emergency treatment in Botswana involved people who were affected by alcohol, and he notes that this was unexpected in the light of previous information in Africa, which suggested physical illness could be more prominent a precursor of acutely disturbed behaviour.

With regard to South Africa, Parry & Bennetts (in press) review a number of studies which show high rates of risky drinking, as carefully defined. According to their review, up to 49 per cent of university students and around 30 per cent of male and over 10 per cent of female high school students admitted to having had at least five drinks in the five days prior to being interviewed. The studies referred to took place in the Western Cape. For adults, the figures may be comparable: a national study cited by Parry and Bennetts (in press) puts the rate of risky drinking at above 30 per cent for African men in South Africa, and at around 20 per cent for African women (Rocha-Silva, 1991). As Rocha-Silva (1997) notes, there is an ongoing increase in alcohol misuse by women. Parry (in press) indicates that drinking patterns amongst youth do not appear to differ substantially across 'racial' lines for males, but a Cape Town study shows lower rates of alcohol use amongst Xhosa-speaking adolescent females than for other females (Flisher et al., 1993a). Rocha-Silva et al. (1995), cited by Parry (in press), claim there is an increase in alcohol intake by adults in South Africa, with particularly marked increases being shown amongst historically disadvantaged Africans and amongst women.

Other drugs

Cocaine and heroin use are associated with a range of undesirable outcomes, including 'death from overdose, infection, violence, AIDS, and circulatory, respiratory, and digestive diseases' (Desjarlais et al., 1995: 97). Internationally, there has been a marked increase in cocaine and heroin abuse, a factor which is made all the more serious with the risks for HIV infection (Oppenheimer, 1991). Because of their different effects on mood, cocaine and heroin are often taken together or as part of a broader pattern of multi-drug use.

Inhalants such as glue, paint thinners, and shoe dye are commonly used and associated with social problems amongst youth. Over 30 per cent of people aged 14-24 in Mexico use inhalants on a regular basis, with children as young as 5 or 6 beginning to use them (Desjarlais et al., 1995: 99). In Brazil, rates of solvent use amongst street youth have been reported to range from 21.5 per cent to 43.5 per cent (Silva-Fihlo et al., 1990, as quoted by Ball & Howard, 1995: 139).

Cannabis (marijuana, dagga) is used widely in many parts of the world, and there is considerable debate as to whether, and to what extent, it is harmful. The question of toxic psychosis following cannabis abuse is an especially interesting one from a cultural perspective, and I shall deal with this issue in a later section.

Prescribed drugs represent a relatively new area of concern. During the 1970s, Librium and Valium (both benzodiazepine drugs – otherwise known as minor tranquillizers) were the most widely prescribed drugs in the world (Ray, 1991; cited by Doyal, 1995: 182). Benzodiazepines have been prescribed far more for women than for men (Doyal, 1995). It has been estimated that in Europe and the USA, approximately 2 to 3 per cent of people are long-term tranquilliser users (Williams & Bellantuono, 1991: 72). The antidepressant Prozac has made psychotropic drugs more visible internationally. By 1990, two years after it had been released in the USA, sales had reached US$350 million, 'more than the combined amount spent on all types of antidepressants before Prozac came on the market'. By 1994, 11 million people world-wide were taking Prozac (figures cited by Lyon, 1996: 58).

Less information is available about the use of drugs in South Africa than about alcohol. Reviewing a series of studies, Parry (in press) notes rates of use of cannabis of up to 22 per cent amongst African males in informal settlements, with usage of LSD and cocaine being almost as high amongst males in towns. For African females, rates of about 10 per cent have been recorded for cocaine and LSD use.

Tobacco

The effects of tobacco on health are well known. It is estimated that the annual cost of morbidity from smoking costs in the region of US$27 billion (figures cited by Helman, 1994: 215). Smoking rates among men have begun to level off internationally, but there is a continuing increase in smoking amongst women, with particular concern about younger smokers in developing countries (Doyal, 1995: 188-191; Helman, 1994: 215; Nichter & Cartwright, 1991). A significant proportion of South Africans smoke, and continue to smoke in spite of knowing about the ill effects (Hirschowitz & Orkin, 1995: 55-56; Martin et al., 1992). Although smoking is a major public health issue in which mental health workers are, and should be, involved, I will not be discussing smoking in this chapter, as space in this book does not permit a broad discussion of cultural factors in health issues (see, though, Dasen et al., 1988; Helman, 1994).

Drugs in cultural context

How the body responds to drugs (prescribed or not) and alcohol may at first glance seem to be purely a matter of physiology. This is, however, not the case, as the following quotation demonstrates:

When a man lifts a cup, it is not only the kind of drink that is in it, the amount he is likely to take, and the circumstances under which he will do the drinking that are specified in advance for him, but also whether the contents of the cup will cheer or stupefy, whether they will induce affection or aggression, quiet or unalloyed pleasure. These and many other cultural definitions attach to the drink even before it reaches the lips. (Mandelbaum, 1965: 282, as quoted by McDonald, 1994: 12)

The above quotation is equally true for women, and McDonald goes on to stress that all substances which affect people's states of mind and which are potentially addictive have their effects in a cultural context. 'Personality, social or cultural backgrounds' (Helman, 1994: 194) have profound effects on responses to prescribed medication and to other substances. It is also true that what is socially defined as an alcohol problem, for example, differs across cultures (Gureje et al., 1997). Expanding on the work of Claridge (1970), Helman (1994) suggests that in understanding the effect of any drug, we need to consider five factors:

1 The attributes of the *drug* itself (such as taste, shape, colour, etc.)
2 The attributes of the *recipient* (such as age, background, personality, etc.)
3 The attributes of the *prescriber* (such as age, professional status, authority, etc.)
4 The physical *setting* in which the drug is prescribed (such as clinic, hospital, social setting, etc.)
5 The *macro-context* in which the above takes place (such as the moral and cultural values attached to the drug, whether the drug is socially valued or disapproved of, whether the drug is taken as part of a cult or family ritual, etc.) (Adapted from Helman, 1994: 194-195)

As is well known in both clinical and lay circles, it is possible to induce drug-like reactions in persons who have taken something which only physically resembles the drug but has none of its chemical properties – this is known as the placebo effect. Clinical trials of pharmacological agents often make use of a research strategy in which some respondents are given the active drug and some a placebo, so that researchers can try to separate out the chemical from the psychosocial effects of the drug. In practice, though, all drug-taking, legal and illegal, prescribed or not, occurs in a sociocultural context. Drug effects cross other boundaries: throughout the world, and this is a well-documented feature of developing countries, people will take drugs prescribed by the informal and folk sectors, as well as those prescribed by professionals, at the same time as taking drugs for their recreational or mood-altering properties (Van der Geest & Whyte, 1988).

The psychology of drug and alcohol use is complex, with a range of factors exerting a strong influence, including the power of the person prescribing or selling a drug, and cultural factors surrounding drug and alcohol use. Gender roles play a major part in determining patterns of usage and abuse. In some areas of Cape Town, for example, it is estimated informally that over 70 per cent of males use dagga, mandrax (methaqualone), or both, a figure which is not altogether out of keeping with scientific data (Flisher et al., 1993b; Rottanburg, 1982; Rottanburg et al., 1982). By contrast, the fact that most people who take overdoses of prescribed drugs are women has been related to issues in gender relationships, and the role of pharmaceutical companies in targeting women in advertising (Littlewood, 1994; Prather, 1991). Ideas about what drugs like tranquillizers can do for people relate strongly to broader social concerns and beliefs about how society is organized, and the way society deals with its difficulties and problems (Montagne, 1991). Ray (1991) emphasizes the role of the political economy and the influence of the global market in pharmaceuticals in contributing to high rates of tranquillizer use. Patterns of drinking and drug-taking may change across time, and the same patterns may come to be described in different ways according to changing cultural norms and values (Orford, 1985; Helman, 1994). The need to understand cultural factors in patterns of drug-taking, and for purposes of treatment, is well established (Akyeampong, 1995; Brown et al., 1993; Dinges & Duong-Tran, 1993; Pena & Koss-Chioino, 1992). Any intervention plan which focuses purely on individuals and does not take into account the social and cultural roles involved in the use and abuse of substances is unlikely to succeed (Desjarlais et al., 1995).

Religious and spiritual beliefs may play a part in patterns of substance use. Dagga plays an important part in Rastafarian ideology and beliefs. Religious groups tend to be quite specific as to which drugs are acceptable. For example, although wine has sacramental functions amongst Jews and Christians, other drugs tend to be frowned upon in these groups. By contrast, Islam forbids the use of alcohol. The drug *qat* (*tchat*; *khat*), however, known as the 'flower of paradise' (Kennedy, 1987), which is used in Ethiopia, Yemen, and other countries in East Africa and the Middle East is 'considered "holy" by devout Muslims' (Almedom & Abraham, 1994: 249).

The debates concerning the physical ill-effects of *qat* also underline cultural issues. A number of biomedical studies have suggested that chewing *qat* may be harmful, resulting in a range of symptoms, including lower birthweight amongst babies born to female chewers. More anthropologically-oriented research, however, has raised questions about how widespread negative health consequences may be (see Almedon & Abraham, 1994, for a review of studies). Almedon and Abraham emphasize the need for biologically-oriented drug research, looking for biological consequences of drug use, to consider the role of cultural assumptions in the formation of questions about these consequences. A number of studies have suggested that *qat* may precipitate psychosis (Desjarlais et al., 1995: 101), though Asuni et al. (1994: 161) suggest that 'mental instability' is a prerequisite for the precipitation of *qat* psychosis. The debates for the existence or otherwise of a *qat*-induced or *qat*-precipitated psychosis are similar to those about 'cannabis psychosis', and we shall now consider some aspects of the cultural construction of cannabis psychosis.

The cultural construction of cannabis psychosis

The DSM-IV makes the following allowance for psychosis associated with cannabis use:

> Psychotic Disorders can occur in association with **intoxication** with the following classes of substances: alcohol; amphetamine and related substances; cannabis; cocaine; hallucinogens; inhalants; opioids (meperidine); phencyclidine and related substances; sedatives, hypnotics, and anxiolytics; and other or unknown substances.

Cannabis-Induced Psychotic Disorder may develop shortly after cannabis use and usually involves persecutory delusions. The disorder is apparently rare. Marked anxiety, emotional lability, depersonalization, and subsequent amnesia for the episode can occur. The disorder usually remits within a day, but in some cases may persist for a few days. Hallucinations associated with Cannabis Intoxication are rare except when very high blood levels are reached. (DSM-IV, 1994: 312)

This picture is of cannabis as rarely having a psychotic outcome, and of the consequences being fairly short-lived. A different view seems to be widely held in Africa, where cannabis psychosis is seen to be common, accounting for a substantial proportion of hospital admissions, and not necessarily having a benign picture (Desjarlais et al., 1995: 100). The following cautionary note is sounded:

Cannabis is not the innocent drug it is sometimes believed to be, and it may precipitate a psychosis on first exposure. (Asuni et al., 1994: 161)

Rottanburg and her colleagues (Rottanburg, 1982; Rottanburg et al., 1982) have suggested that there may be a psychosis with manic features following cannabis use (they are careful not to claim explicitly a cannabis-*induced* psychosis, but this is an implication of the line of their research). Psychiatrists in training in Cape Town believed that cannabis was responsible for a proportion of admissions to a psychiatric hospital (Swartz, 1989). Statistics from a psychiatric emergency unit in Cape Town, for a few months in 1988, revealed that 'substance induced organic brain syndrome' was the second most common diagnosis made, along with schizophrenia and major depression.

There are many problems in trying to delineate the existence or otherwise of a cannabis-induced psychosis. Rottanburg (1982) found cannabinoids (chemical evidence of dagga usage) in the urine of a substantial proportion of patients in a South African psychiatric hospital. If, however, dagga use is as widespread as it appears to be (Flisher et al., 1993b), then one would expect to find cannabinoids in the urine of many people who are *not* in a psychiatric hospital, and one would need to show a significantly higher rate of cannabinoids in the hospital group in order to demonstrate dagga as a risk factor for being in hospital. It is also difficult to separate out the potential effects of dagga from those of other drugs used, when it is clear that multiple drugs, including alcohol, may be used by certain groups. Claims for dagga's being responsible for psychosis may also be affected by beliefs within the group of people who are diagnosing. Swartz (1989) showed that talk of 'toxic psychosis' following dagga use on the part of clinicians operated in a similar way to talk of culture as an issue in diagnosis. Sumba (1991) suggests there may also be a problem, in talk of the effects of cannabis, of confusing cause with effect – 'heavy cannabis use could be a result of deviance rather than its cause' (Sumba, 1991: 344).

The most outspoken discussion of how the label 'toxic psychosis' or 'cannabis psychosis' can have social underpinnings comes from Britain. Littlewood (1988) has described the use of the label 'cannabis psychosis' in an apparently racist way in Birmingham. Community workers felt that the diagnosis was being used to obtain involuntary admission for black men to psychiatric institutions. Birmingham psychiatrists, in spite of being unable to agree on the existence or diagnostic picture of 'cannabis psychosis', were making the diagnosis consistently, and dramatically more often, for black patients than for white and, Littlewood and Lipsedge (1997) point out, in the absence of evidence of cannabinoids being found in the patients' urine (McGovern & Cope, 1987). A leading article by Littlewood and Lipsedge (1988) in the *British Medical Journal*, which reported, amongst other things, on the 'cannabis psychosis' issue, drew the response from two Birmingham psychiatrists that cannabis psychosis does not appear as a diagnosis in their current ongoing study of admissions (Milner & Hayes, 1988). Littlewood and Lipsedge interpret this change from the findings of McGovern and Cope (1987) as follows:

A heavily publicized survey of local psychiatrists' attitudes showed that there was little general agreement on whether 'cannabis psychosis' existed and what its symptoms might be (Littlewood, 1988) ... Attempts to have a joint psychiatrists/

community workers meeting were unsuccessful but one possible consequence was that the diagnosis suddenly disappeared locally (Milner & Hayes, 1988). (Littlewood & Lipsedge, 1997: 276)

Clearly, Littlewood and Lipsedge are claiming that racial factors may affect the use of a diagnosis like 'cannabis psychosis'. South African psychiatrists in training, in a study of their responses to clinical vignettes, tended to suggest a 'toxic psychosis' diagnosis less often amongst vignettes designated as being about black 'African' patients than about others (Swartz, 1989). This may reflect a desire on the part of these clinicians, at a time when political violence in South Africa was at a high level, not to succumb to racist diagnostic practices. Whatever the reason, it appears that in both Britain and South Africa, ideas about race and ideas about drugs like cannabis interact in the kinds of decisions clinicians may make affecting patients. The 'cannabis psychosis' debate, then, helps us realize that we must understand not only that drug effects are powerfully affected by non-pharmacological factors. We must also understand that claims made by professionals about the effects of drugs (harmful or otherwise) may also be affected by cultural factors and by the beliefs of professionals about drugs, and about who use drugs and why.

Some concluding thoughts on alcohol, drugs, and culture

The widespread use of drugs all over the world poses some difficulties for us when we attempt to study mental illness in its 'pure' (drug-free) form. The fact that drugs of various kinds, legal and illegal, are used so widely, means that in practice the 'pure' mental illness unaffected by drug use is far less common than a neatly-ordered view of the world would have us believe. As we have also seen, we cannot view drugs, furthermore, as purely pharmacological agents, as a range of cultural and personal factors will shape the effects of drug usage. Cultural factors will also shape professionals' beliefs about the effects, good or bad, of both prescribed and non-prescribed drugs. Cultural (and racist) stereotypes about which groups are more or less likely to abuse drugs will also affect the way professionals think (Howitt & Owusu-Bempah, 1994: 134-135).

Thinking about drugs in a holistic way, which does not deny the pharmacological effects of drugs but puts these effects in a broader context, can help us plan interventions more sensitively. Unless we know the social meanings of drugs and people's theories about how they affect their lives (Fainzang, 1996), we will not be able to help people in the best way possible. The cultural study of drug use spans the boundaries of biology and psychology, physiology and culture. In the following section, we shall see how the concept of dissociation also raises interesting questions about the categories we use in the field of culture and mental health.

Dissociation in cultural perspective

According to the DSM-IV,

> [t]he essential feature of the Dissociative Disorders is a dis-ruption in the usually integrated functions of consciousness, memory, identity, or perception of the environment. The disturbance may be sudden or gradual, transient or chronic. (DSM-IV, 1994: 477)

Castillo (1997: 219) notes that trance is a central part of dissociation. Trance is a 'narrowed focus of attention, such that what is outside of attention is lost to consciousness' (Castillo, 1997: 219). According to the DSM-IV(1994: 477), there are four central dissociative states. Dissociative amnesia involves the inability to remember important personal information, usually of a traumatic or stressful nature (the amnesia goes beyond ordinary forgetfulness). Dissociative fugue involves sudden travel away from home, inability to remember the past, and either the assumption of a new identity or confusion about past identity. Dissociative identity disorder (formerly known as Multiple Personality Disorder) occurs when there are two or more distinct personalities which take control of the person's behaviour, together with features of amnesia. Depersonalization disorder consists of a feeling of being detached from mental or bodily processes, while at the same time being in touch with reality.

As we have seen earlier, PTSD may also include dissociative symptoms, as may other disorders. The DSM-IV notes that

> [a] cross-cultural perspective is particularly important in the evaluation of Dissociative Disorders because dissociative states are a common and accepted expression of cultural activities or religious experience in many societies. Dissociation should not be considered inherently pathological and often does not lead to significant distress, impairment, or help-seeking behavior. However, a number of culturally defined syndromes characterized by dissociation do cause distress and impairment and are recognized indigenously as manifestations of pathology. (DSM-IV, 1994: 477)

Part of the difficulty in studying dissociation lies precisely in the fact that dissociation is not 'inherently pathological' as the DSM-IV puts it (above). It is not always easy to distinguish between what is an 'acceptable' form of dissociation and an 'unacceptable' form (Putnam, 1993), a factor which is further complicated when one is looking at dissociation cross-culturally. Another factor affecting how we think about dissociation is the degree of controversy surrounding the area. Hacking (1995) opens his study of multiple personality, much of it devoted to questions surrounding the cultural construction of the disorder, with a chapter entitled 'Is it real?' In this chapter, he shows that the debates surrounding the existence of multiple personality disorder have been fierce over the past decade. At the same time, though,

> dissociative disorders are the current 'rage' in the psychological and psychiatric communities. Indeed, interest in dissociative disorders has increased exponentially in the last decade or so, and harkens back to the prominence dissociative phenomena enjoyed in the field of psychology more than 100 years ago. (Lynn & Rhue, 1994: 1)

An interesting cultural question is why there is such a resurgence of interest in dissociation at present. Is it simply that there is now an 'epidemic' of dissociative disorders in the West and, if so, why? Could it be that dissociative disorders are now being discovered because we are for the first time looking for them properly? Were we, for most of this century, relatively blind to dissociative disorders, which were there all along? Is there perhaps something about dissociative disorders which 'speaks' to us now, towards the end of this century, which makes them the focus of so much attention now? Is the continuity between 'normal' and 'abnormal' dissociation part of what makes dissociative disorders so interesting to clinicians?

These are all interesting cultural hypotheses. Another question is that of how the cross-cultural literature on what appears to be dissociation can help us understand dissociation in general. Castillo (1994a, 1994b) argues that dissociation may play an important part in spirit possession as seen in South Asia (and, by implication, in Africa, as we have seen in previous chapters). Certainly, trance phenomena, and some features of what are known as culture-bound syndromes (see Chapter 7) do seem to have a possession component. Central to Castillo's (1994b) understanding of dissociation in spirit possession is the idea that a traumatic event or experience is a precipitant of dissociation. He argues further that

> [e]vidence suggests that pathological spirit possession in India, and multiple personality disorder in North America are psycho-culturally distinct but parallel trance-related disorders, that is, manifestations of the same underlying pathogenic process, experienced, expressed, and understood in culturally specific cognitive categories. (Castillo, 1994b: 141)

Other culture-bound syndromes such as *amafufunyana*, for example, as classically described by Ngubane (see Chapter 7), could also be understood in terms of dissociation. The foreign voices with which the person speaks could be seen as dissociated and separated from the rest of consciousness. Similar arguments could be made for *ukuthwasa*, which could be seen as a more positive possession state. If this is the case, should we be looking for traumatic precipitants for possession syndromes, as Castillo (1994b) does in his reinterpretation of South Asian spirit possession? And can the florid nature of many culture-bound syndromes provide models for understanding dissociative disorders in dominant culture?

Certainly, much of the resurgence of clinical interest in dissociation is associated with the enormous emphasis in the media, amongst professionals, and in society more broadly, on trauma and abuse (Belli & Loftus, 1994; Glass, 1993; Spiegel, 1993a). As we have seen in Chapter 8 in relation to PTSD, we cannot simply assume that an increase in discussion of trauma means that there is definitely an increase in trauma, or even that trauma that was formerly hidden is now being discovered. Levett (1988) has shown how the ways we speak about childhood sexual abuse, for example, relates partly to other concerns and power relationships in the society. She suggests further that one effect of being seen as a survivor of sexual abuse is not, as one might expect, concern for the survivor's well-being but, instead, stigmatization – an example of what she refers to as the 'violence of representation' (Levett, 1995). In studying talk about child sexual abuse amongst black South African women, Levett et al. (1997) found they had to confront assumptions commonly held by professionals about the nature of abuse and its effects, as these assumptions often did not make sense to the respondents. In looking for the effects of abuse, therefore, the 'symptoms' for which we search may be cultural explanations of and prescriptions for life after abuse, and not value-free entities which are waiting to be discovered. In the light of this kind of information, it is not surprising that Tillman et al. (1994) problematize the relationship between trauma and dissociative pathology, arguing that simplistic notions of cause and effect are not sufficient. They point out that there may be a tendency to underemphasize the evidence of dissociation occurring in the absence of trauma, and of trauma not leading to dissociation, and to overemphasize data which links dissociation to trauma (Tillman et al., 1994: 409). Part of the reason for this tendency may rest with the kinds of cultural assumptions we hold about dissociation and trauma.

As we have seen in Chapter 7, one of the major challenges in understanding culture-bound syndromes is to think about how culture-bound syndromes comment on and reflect central concerns about the contexts in which they occur. If dissociative disorders in dominant culture have something in common with many aspects of culture-bound syndromes, perhaps we need to ask similar questions about the new 'epidemic' of dissociation. For many years in this century dissociation received very little clinical attention except in the cross-cultural literature. In this respect, dissociation was to some degree associated with thinking about 'non-Western' people, and with images of the primitive. Evolutionist theories of cultural development and difference, furthermore, portrayed the Western ideal of the autonomous individual as superior to other cultural norms. These include notions in other societies which depend more on an appreciation of how people change in different contexts. Within a sociocentric approach to understanding people, identities may depend on group and local definitions (Shweder & Bourne, 1982). Modernization theory held that there was a progression from 'premodern' ways of being to a more autonomous, individualized view of the world which emphasizes scientific rationality and personal agency in the world (Inkeles & Smith, 1974). The journey of modernization was portrayed as essentially in one direction – towards the better state of being as a modern, autonomous individual. This view holds potential for problems of ethnocentrism (Castillo, 1997), which may be especially problematic in racially divided societies like apartheid South Africa (Swartz, 1985b). It also allows us to think of possession states and dissociation as a whole as products of 'primitive' cultures which believe in 'non-scientific' things such as superstition and witchcraft.

It has by now been well proved that 'magical' or superstitious thinking, thought to be a product of the less developed world, is found universally (Shweder, 1977, 1984). Beliefs in 'science', greatly valued in Western culture, are not necessarily based on any more personal evidence than are beliefs in spiritual forces in other cultures, and there is increasing recognition that non-rational factors play a part in the development of science as well as in other areas of endeavour (Gilbert & Mulkay, 1984). The neat divisions of the modern versus the premodern world simply do not hold.

The questioning of modernity as the end point of cultural

evolution goes much further, however. The world with which we are confronted at present is different from what the 'modern' world seemed to be at one time. Fast, efficient modes of travel and improved communications coupled with many civil and guerrilla wars have led to migrations on an unprecedented scale. This is occurring to the extent that anthropologists are increasingly trying to understand culture without the assumption that cultures are bounded in either time or place (Olwig & Hastrup, 1997). It is also becoming clear that apparently culture-free 'givens' such as 'place' and 'space' are in fact areas of huge conflict of interpretation (Dixon, 1997; Dixon et al., 1994; Ramphele, 1993). In addition, the very technologies that encourage physical movements across the world also permit movements of a more abstract kind. In writing this book in Cape Town, South Africa, for example, I have spent a considerable amount of time 'surfing' the Internet, 'visiting' sites dealing with culture and mental health in many different parts of the world. Turkle (1995) has shown how profound the psychological effects of the Internet can be. The Internet can blur divisions between the 'I' and the 'not-I', allowing people to take on multiple identities and to try out different 'selves'. There are media reports about Internet romances that go disastrously wrong when couples who have fallen in love with identities on the screen (as Turkle would put it) find that the embodied people who created and lived through those identities are not the same as the identities.

The modern idea of the coherent individual – and of coherent culture – is fragmenting and changing (Bibeau, 1997). The science fiction film *Strange days* depicts an end of the twentieth century culture in which it has become possible through technology to have access to, and to replay, the actual experiences of other people – to experience fully their internal, visceral responses to the world. Although this is fiction, it speaks of the concerns of late twentieth century society in which the world is more fragmented yet more accessible. Even the boundaries of the body no longer encapsulate the 'self' adequately any more – both because of computer technology and because of transplants and spare-part surgery (Helman, 1991). In this context, and in the context of great strides in artificial intelligence, the boundaries between human and technological identity, between what is a person and what is a machine are increasingly blurred (Turkle, 1995).

Violence and coercion are also features of the world:

> [T]he end of the twentieth century is a bloody time ... The suffering that results from political violence includes a range of traumas: pain, anguish, fear, loss, grief, and *the destruction of a coherent and meaningful reality*. (Kleinman, 1995b: 174, emphasis added)

Technology enables images of violence to be produced easily and instantly, such that what may be termed the fragmentation of belief associated with mass violence becomes part of reality throughout the world. Millions of people who have never seen, and never will see Soweto, Ethiopia, Tiananmen Square in Beijing, and Bosnia have a sense of the look and the sound of such places at times of violence and terror (Kleinman & Kleinman, 1996). Hostage-taking, which can occur in conflicts running the gamut from domestic dispute to international hostility, has profound implications for the sense of enduring identity on the part of hostages and, probably, of the hostage-takers themselves (Lipsedge & Littlewood, 1997; West & Martin, 1994). Hostage dramas are also part of the news all over the world. There is also an upsurge of interest in, and talk about, cults which have a profound effect on how we think about identity and what it means to be human. Some cults are very much in the public eye, partly because of the apparently willing participation of large groups of people in their own destruction – the Guyana of Jim Jones, Waco in Texas, and even the comet Hale-Bopp are all places familiar to the late twentieth century person who follows the media. Debate about satanism, satanist abuse, and other ritual and cult-based abuses has never been stronger (Sinason, 1994; Spanos & Burgess, 1994), and media interest in satanism is such that in the late 1980s 'Satan had become the star of American television talk shows' (Hacking, 1995: 114). Hacking describes shows like those of Geraldo Rivera and Oprah Winfrey as 'the circuses of our days' (Hacking, 1995: 36), and in these 'circuses', watched by millions of people all over the world, devil possession, satanic cults, and multiple personality form part of the entertainment.

Part of the fascination leading to an explosion of interest in abuse, possession, and dissociation has been the inversion of power. The abused are encouraged to speak out against authority figures, to accuse such figures (including their parents) of terrible, inhumane deeds. In response to what some have seen as a situation of witch-hunts similar to those depicted so vividly in Arthur Miller's play *The crucible*, questions have been raised as to the accuracy of allegations made. In 1992, the False Memory Syndrome Foundation was established to support parents accused of abuse by their children:

> It accuses gullible clinicians, including those who work with multiple personality, of generating memories that never happened. In return, activists on the other side say that the foundation is a support group for child abusers. (Hacking, 1995: 14)

In the public arena, the very concept of memory is being questioned and disputed (Sinason, in press). Clinicians and researchers have long known that perfect recall is an impossibility, and that many contextual factors shape how we view our past. But when there is widespread bitter public debate about whose memories in a family are 'true' and whose 'false', this raises questions in the broader community about the continuity of consciousness and of the ways we organize our lives psychologically.

In the context of this world, a sense of fragmentation may be not only possible, but normative. Social scientists have for some time been thinking differently about how we should understand people. The notion of the 'fixed' personality, central to much psychiatric thinking, can no longer be taken for granted, as we emphasize more and more how people, and their senses of themselves, can change under changing circumstances (Henriques et al., 1984). When Spiegel (1993b) introduces a text on dissociative disorders with the sentence 'Unity of consciousness is an achievement, not a given' (Spiegel, 1993b: ix), he does this in the context of a world in which there is increasing emphasis on fragmentation not only as a normal part of how people live their lives, but also as a basis for under standing people:

> [P]ost-structuralism proposes a subjectivity which is precarious, contradictory and in process, constantly being constituted in discourse each time we think or speak. (Weedon, 1987: 32-33, as quoted by Mama, 1995)

Postmodernism, a theory strongly linked to post-structuralism,

> is a philosophy that has reacted strongly against several assumptions of modernity: those concerning progress, history, causality, system, absolutes, meaning, the unitary self, technological judgement, and conformity. It celebrates difference, change, transformation and flux. (Glass, 1993: 1)

Postmodernism thrives on ideas about plurality of experience, and multiple interpretation. Identity, rather than being fixed, is constantly being negotiated and redefined within a matrix of power relationships – what postmodernists term the 'unitary subject' (Glass, 1993: 6) is critiqued and said to no longer exist. Culture, similarly, becomes 'a contested space' (Jordan & Weedon, 1995: 8). Discussions rage about which 'truth' we should accept and who has the authority to claim knowledge of, and speak about, the world. In contradistinction to what have been termed 'hegemonic' voices, and voices of the colonizers having authority about what is and is not said about the world, there is interest in 'subaltern' voices – voices of women, of the formerly colonized, of sexual and racial minorities, for example, now being allowed to speak (Jordan & Weedon, 1995; Spivak, 1990). Reality itself is contested, as there are so many interpretations of it. This occurs to the extent that Hacking finds it necessary to say the following early in his book:

> There is a current fashion, among intellectuals who identify themselves as postmodern, to surround the word *reality* with a shower of ironical quotation marks. That is not my fashion. I do not use scare-quotes, and I am not ironical about reality. (Hacking, 1995: 16)

Postmodernism as a critical movement can be criticized further for the way it sets itself up as having a privileged view of the world, in spite of its overt commitment to plurality of views. The important point for our discussion, though, is that our world is being seen as fragmented and volatile. Our knowledge of it comes through images which are endlessly reproduced and changed – the pop music video, for example, thrives on the use of computer-generated methods which can reproduce images and change them endlessly and believably. We cannot be sure whether photographs we see in the newspapers are 'real' images, or whether they have been changed through computer technology. Power relationships which were once well entrenched are being questioned and changed. Social scientists are seeing identity as fragmented and reality as negotiable and questionable. This is an ideal context in which dissociative disorders should be fascinating. Like culture-bound syndromes, as generally understood, they encapsulate in heightened form many of our current anxieties and preoccupations about the world. Whereas even ten years ago it was possible to think of dissociation as typically something associated with 'the primitive', this is no longer the case. Spirit possession, bewitchment, fugues, and trances, once seen as features of 'premodern' societies, are postmodern phenomena as well. To be possessed, as we reach the end of this century, is to be a person of our times. The old dualistic distinctions between the 'developed' and the 'undeveloped', the 'civilized' and the 'uncivilized' will no longer hold – and it is, in part, the phenomenon of dissociation which is making this clear to us. Throughout this book I have suggested that it is a mistake to see the cultural study of mental health and illness as the study of the 'other', or the 'primitive'. The rise in interest in dissociative disorders in dominant Western culture makes it clear that cultural issues in mental health should not be seen as at the fringes of dominant culture, but at the centre.

Concluding comments

This chapter has dealt with three areas which question some assumptions about culture and mental health. The literature on transient psychosis leads us to question universalist categories of serious mental disorder, and also to think about the interweaving of biological and psychocultural issues in precipitating mental disorder. Thinking about alcohol and drugs helps us to consider more closely the combined effects of biological and psychosocial variables on human emotions and behaviour. From a cultural perspective, furthermore, it is possible to think about legal and illegal drugs, and drugs that are biomedically prescribed and those that are not, in similar ways. The extent of drug use leads us to place in cultural context our desire to isolate and understand 'pure' mental disorders which are free from the influence of drugs. We find ourselves constantly crossing back and forth across the boundaries from the 'mental' to the 'physiological' or 'somatic', and come to realize that these boundaries are possibly more of our own making than existing 'out there' in the world. The increasing interest in dissociation links disorders commonly seen as disorders of 'primitive' people with those disorders which are the object of intense debate and scrutiny in the Western world at present. Dissociation, so much a feature of what have been seen as 'traditional' illnesses, is equally a feature of the way many of us live our lives now. What we might once have thought about as a fairly clear distinction between the 'primitive' and the 'developed' person, in the face of this cultural shift, becomes more and more difficult to see – in fact, it may not be there at all!

The fact that there is so much to learn in terms of mental health practice from phenomena and debates at what I have termed the borderland makes this a very exciting place to be thinking about. The breaking up of old boundaries and the questioning of truths about mental health and illness all have implications for how we work together in the mental health field. This will be discussed in the following chapter.

PART IV

Conclusion

11

Working together

In this concluding chapter we shall consider some of the implications of what we have learned thus far for how we work to improve mental health and to reduce the burden of mental illness. It is clear that, although mental health issues have been identified as a priority in the 1993 World Bank report *Investing in health*, much remains to be done to ensure that these issues are addressed adequately in national and international programmes (Blue & Harpham, 1994; Desjarlais et al., 1995: 259). A key point to recognize is that mental health challenges cannot be separated from other health and social issues, and that the distinctions we make between mental health and other issues often have to do with convenience, or with cultural factors in the construction of different disciplines.

One of our central tasks, if we apply a cultural understanding of mental health issues, is to recognize the interrelatedness and importance of intervening with these issues in a multi-pronged manner. Poverty, discrimination, and political oppression are all implicated in mental health problems. At the same time, biological factors have been shown to play a part in serious and minor mental disorder. Political and economic empowerment programmes, as well as biological interventions, though, can all fail if due attention is not given to cultural and local social factors. Having a cultural understanding of mental health issues does not mean having to choose between, say, economic analyses and biological understandings of mental health and disorder. On the contrary, it implies an approach which can in form a diverse range of skills and interventions. But how do we orchestrate everything that is needed? This is a difficult question to answer, and full treatment of it would require much longer than a chapter in a book. What we can do here, though, is to think about some of the lessons that a cultural understanding can give us towards reaching the ambitious goal of better mental health for all. Broad policy is clearly important, and will be dealt with later, but it is useful to begin with a consideration of some of the issues involved in working together even at the most local level.

Many disciplines, one aim?

As we have seen throughout this book, there are many views on mental health issues. Some of them work together in a comple- mentary fashion, and some conflict with one another. It has become a truism that 'modern psychiatry is unthinkable without the multi- disciplinary team' (Gillis, 1986a: 228). The multidisciplinary team may consist of a variety of professionals, depending on context. These may include medical practitioners (including psychiatrists), psychologists, social workers, occupational therapists, psychiatric nurses, and sometimes other professionals including other psychotherapists who may, for example, be psychoanalytically trained. Although this team is there to attend to the patients' needs in complementary ways, there is potential for conflict amongst the different groups. Some of this conflict may relate to the power relationships between professions, and the fact that often, for very similar work, members of different professions earn vastly different amounts of money. Skirmishes over boundaries of disciplinary competence may arise, some of which have to do with the fact that a profession is constructed culturally to have sole expertise over a single area, and it becomes a problem when there are competing claims for competence in a narrow field (Abbott, 1988).

It is within the general health field that professionals see the great- est number of mental health problems, with formal mental health services seeing only a proportion of these problems (Goldberg & Huxley, 1980; 1992). Within the health field, mental health profes- sionals are granted the status of 'experts' over the realm of the emotions. Miller and Swartz (1990b, 1991) have shown how the presence of mental health professionals in such settings can complicate rather than improve health care. They tell of a case of a boy who was admitted to a neurosurgery ward in Cape Town (Miller & Swartz, 1991). Staff on the ward were concerned that the boy was depressed, and they arranged for him to be seen by a clinical psychologist, so his depression could be properly assessed and he could possibly be placed on antidepressant medication. The psychologist went to see the boy and, as she could not speak his language (Xhosa), she asked a member of the nursing staff to interpret. The first thing the boy said was that he needed to pass water. He could not converse with most of the staff, and had been lying in bed feeling very uncomfortable. It emerged on interview that the boy was far away from home and his family, and was in an environment where few people could speak his language. He felt lonely and homesick. Those nursing staff who could speak with him were busy with nursing duties and did not see chatting with patients as part of their job. The solution to the boy's 'depression' was to arrange that someone did chat with him regularly. The 'depression' lifted. There is no doubt that the intervention of the psychologist was useful in this case, but the case raises a number of questions. What was essentially a problem of inadequate language resources on the part of the hospital rapidly became, to the ward personnel, a problem of the patient. This problem, further, was turned into the 'disease' of depression. Had a psychologist with a different approach been assigned to the ward, there is even the possibility that antidepressants might well have been prescribed. But what if there had been no psychologist? It is possible that a decision to put the boy on antidepressants might have been made by the medical staff (who do not need to consult a mental health professional in order to prescribe such medicines). But it is also possible that in the absence of an 'expert' who can claim the field of emotional distress as professional territory, other staff might have been able to think and speak more freely about something rather obvious that was troubling the boy. Paradoxically, the presence of the psychologist may have made these people less able to deal with emotional issues as they could have been intimidated and silenced by the psychologist's apparently superior knowledge.

There are many other possible interpretations of what happened in this case. Professional, interprofessional, gender, and race politics may all have played a part in the silence of the Xhosa-speaking staff with respect to the needs of the patient, and their not being able to spend time with him. The important point for our discussion, though, is that having members of different professions available to patients will not necessarily improve the care. Understanding something about the cultural construction of professions, and the relationships between them, may help us to anticipate some of the problems and to avoid them (Swartz & Miller, 1992b).

One of the issues which has engaged the attention of many social scientists in trying to understand why psychosocial issues are so often marginalized in the health care field is that of the power of medicine as a dominant institution. As we have seen earlier in this book, medicine in the past has worked best by dividing up the body into manageable units and by developing subspecialties (Gordon, 1988; Toulmin, 1978). There have been many attempts to broaden the scope of biomedicine and to focus more on illness experience where appropriate (see, for example, Engel, 1977). Unfortunately, such attempts may not always promote an approach which takes adequate account of the patient's perspective, and may instead transform patient concerns into bits of information easily incorporated into the medical perspective (Armstrong, 1987; Lock & Lella, 1986). Though medical dominance in the health care field is undoubtedly an issue, it is all too easy to get into a situation in which doctors, by virtue of their earning the most money and having the most ascribed power, are attacked for all the shortcomings of health care. Blaming doctors is generally not especially helpful as all it does is to place everyone in a static, and unhappy, position in the hierarchy, and it leaves little room for change in a direction which will assist patients. The issue of medical power, furthermore, is far more complex than was thought at one time, and there are all sorts of threats to medical power and autonomy at present – including the rise of a business or corporate model in the provision of health care, increasing legal challenges to medicine and to individual doctors, and the increasing strength of other health care systems (Eisenberg, 1995; Gabe et al., 1994). Biomedicine has no easy answers for chronic and lifestyle diseases or, at present, for the AIDS epidemic. In this context conventional biomedicine is not as much at centre stage as it once was.

We have seen that multidisciplinary work in mental health care may not always be as simply good for the patient as may appear, but to blame the difficulties on a crude analysis of medical power is also not helpful. Having a culturally informed approach to the issue can help us to understand something of the way professions may work. We also know that members of all professions can easily lose sight of the fact that patients come to us with their own complex and contradictory stories, and these cannot easily or accurately be reduced to small packages, each of which corresponds to the expertise of a particular professional. A culturally informed analysis of health and illness should help us find a way to discuss and think together about what the patient may need (Steinberg, 1992). Interdisciplinary conflict can be a very good thing for patients provided members of different professions have the confidence and power to engage with and influence the views of others. This is not easily achievable in practice, but it is possible (Swartz & Miller, 1992b). It is far more useful to recognize conflict as a potential resource to be mobilized on behalf of the patient than to hope that if conflict is not spoken of, it will disappear.

My argument thus far has focused chiefly on working within teams of professionals, all of whom have expertise in the mental health field. We shall now look at some of the issues we face when working with paraprofessionals or non-professionals in the mental health arena, before looking at the question of intersectoral collaboration.

Training and consultation for culturally appropriate mental health work

There are very few mental health professionals in Africa, as we have seen in Chapter 4 (see also Asuni, 1991; Ben-Tovim, 1987; Mustafa, 1991; Patel & Winston, 1994). We also know that people with mental health problems make use of a range of healing systems, only one of which is biomedicine. It seems to follow logically, then, that if we wish to make a significant impact on mental health in Africa, we need to engage with a variety of resources, and to ensure that appropriate mental health knowledge is spread as widely as possible across a range of helpers. Many projects have tried to do just this. In this section, rather than review a variety of projects, I shall mention some key cultural issues for training and working with nonprofessionals or paraprofessionals. Because of my own experience, and because community health workers are working in the mental health area in a number of South African projects, I shall focus on working with community health workers (CHWs). These I define as people without formal tertiary education who work in their own communities after short training courses given by professionals.

Key issues in working with community health workers

Since the Alma Ata Declaration (WHO, 1978), CHWs have been employed in many countries of the world to help achieve the WHO goal of health for all by the year 2000 (Walt, 1990). There was considerable optimism about the ability of CHWs to realize this goal, and there has also been some disappointment:

> Idealized as a way to overcome many of the limitations of clinic-based medical systems, community health workers (CHWs) were initially hailed as likely to make a major contribution to the success of primary health care initiatives. They were envisioned as being selected by their peers and perhaps even compensated by them, in money or in goods, rather than by governments or international agencies. They were to provide culturally-sensitive preventive and curative care to people – often their own friends and neighbors – who otherwise would have had no easy access to biomedical health services. Sometimes these goals have been realized, but it is also clear that in many parts of the world CHWs have not been allowed to live up to their full potential. (Wood, 1990)

Part of the CHW ideology is that CHWs, coming from the same community as the people they serve, will be in tune with them

culturally and will therefore not experience the same cultural ali-
enation and difficulties experienced by many professionals working
with the community. Though there is much to recommend this view,
there are also significant problems with it. First, it tends to assume that
communities are homogeneous, and to overlook the fact that in all
communities there are differences of opinion, battles for power,
control, and resources, and that no single person (or small group of
people) can be seen to represent the interests of the entire community.
In Chapter 2 we saw some of the difficulties faced by interpreters who
are asked to 'stand for' or act as authorities on the cultural beliefs of
patients. CHWs may experience similar problems.

The fact that CHWs often live in the communities they serve may
well make them closer to the lives of community members, but this
may also present difficulties. Binedell (1991) found CHWs in Cape
Town to be overwhelmed to a degree by their own desire to assist
community members who were living in severe poverty. Community
members would approach them for help at all hours of the day and
night, and they found it difficult to turn people away, especially when
they were hungry and desperate. Pressure such as this, Binedell (1991)
notes, has been argued to contribute to the high burn-out rate and staff
turnover in CHW programmes. Health professions, and mental
health professions in particular, depend partly for their success on a
power differential and some distance between the clinician and the
group served by the clinician. Overlooking the fact that CHWs are
people with privacy needs and needs to get away from work (just like
everyone else) is to see them as part of an Arcadian primitive group,
always in touch with their communities, and always available (cf.
Lucas & Barrett, 1995). Maw (1996), in her work as a mental health
consultant to CHWs, found that one of the important functions she
played was in working against this expectation, and encouraging
CHWs to take time off for themselves and for their own lives

A related problematic assumption about CHWs is that they automatically know about and understand all the mental health problems
of their own community. This again is an unrealistic expectation of
anybody – even of a qualified mental health professional. Binedell
(1993), as we have seen earlier, showed that CHWs tend to know about

socially disruptive mental health problems, but may not know about other, more common, and relatively easily managed difficulties such as depression and anxiety. Training and ongoing support is necessary for these difficulties to be recognized and managed by CHWs.

There may be serious ideological differences between CHWs and professionals, and these can create difficulties. One project I worked on operated in a community where there were many very religious people. One of the CHWs was having marital difficulties and was considering a divorce. This was considered a problem for the project, as CHWs expected that they should set an example to the community, and divorce was frowned upon in the community. At the time, though, one of the team of professionals offering back-up support to the CHWs, but who did not live in the community, was divorced, but this was not considered a problem. I found it difficult to accept that different standards were being applied to community members from those applied to professionals from the outside. A more complex problem was that surrounding homosexuality in the community. Though homosexuality was at one time considered a mental disorder, with changes within European and North American culture, homosexuality is now viewed as a variation rather than an abnormality (see Chapter 3). In the community in which the CHW programme was operating, however, homosexuality was considered a sin and/or a sign of sickness, and there was a widespread perception that any CHW programme with a mental health component would assist in stopping homosexual behaviour in the community. To go along with the community's beliefs in this regard could be seen by some to be the appropriate response of a cultural relativist. In my view, however, a situation such as this calls for taking a position in line with one's own beliefs. In mental health work, one's ultimate clients are often those who are stigmatized and rejected in their own communities, and if one simply goes along with the views of the majority, or the most vocal, in that community, one may lose one's ability to assist those clients. Blumberg et al. (1996) have explored some of the challenges associated with attempting to intervene in wife abuse in a community where CHWs hold different views on the issue than do the professionals from the outside. There are no easy answers to such issues, but the important thing is to recognize the potential for conflict for what it is, and to engage with the conflict. There is, of course, an echo here of my earlier comments on the multidisciplinary team. A cultural understanding of the issues at stake helps us accept that differences in interpretation are to be expected and engaged with, rather than to be avoided.

The content of training and support programmes

How do we train CHWs rapidly and effectively in community mental health work? There is no easy answer to this question. It is clear, though, that although CHWs are often employed to contribute to the prevention of health problems and to health promotion, it is often easier for them to be involved in practical, curative work which is easily visible and measurable (Helman, 1994; Katzenellenbogen et al., 1995; Wood, 1990). For example, it is easier to explain to an outsider how many wounds one has dressed in a day than how one went about preventing mental health problems in the community. Careful qualitative assessment can detect the impact of the 'soft' side of CHW work – the caring, and the listening, for example (Matthews et al., 1994). It is nevertheless tempting to provide CHWs with tangible skills which are easy to see and to measure.

Given this fact, it is hardly surprising that a number of pro grammes which I am familiar with base their training of CHWs on the DSM-IV (1994). CHWs are given a crash course in DSM-IV principles and some of the syndromes. We have seen in Chapter 3 that the DSM-IV holds a central role in the cultural identity of professional mental health workers. But we need to ask how helpful it is in the context of scarce resources for CHWs to be able to diagnose at a very fine level of discrimination. Clearly, the better the assessment that a CHW can do, the more focused a treatment plan can be. When, however, there are few drugs and fewer other forms of therapy on offer, fine-grained diagnostic distinctions may be less important than the CHW's being able to enquire in an empathic way about the person's illness experience. In this regard, a number of programmes now offer basic courses in counselling, which emphasize listening skills and the development of a relationship between the CHW and the client (see, for example, Sterling and Lazarus, 1995).

If CHWs are to be able to support their communities, it is important that they are given sufficient support and ongoing consultation and/or supervision in their work. Maw (1996) found that issues of racial, class, and cultural difference could be discussed openly between her and her consultees only once an ongoing and safe relationship had developed. Establishing such a relationship can take a long time and requires commitment. It is a myth that community work is quick and easy, especially where community work is being used as an attempt to gain a quick understanding of another culture. A good relationship with CHWs, however, can be a profound learning experience for professionals. To say, theoretically, that the area of cultural difference is contested and complex is one thing; to experience these complexities is quite another. Though the frustrations may be great, there is much to be learned, and the experience can be quite exhilarating for all parties.

Intersectoral collaboration

Mental health issues affect, and are affected by, a range of other issues – including health, education, labour, welfare, and gender issues. Mental health needs are ideally met by the best that many sectors can offer. In a community health programme I was involved in, one woman was identified as depressed and was referred to a psychologist for counselling. She found it difficult to engage with the psychologist and did not return for the number of sessions suggested. She discovered, however, that the health programme was also offering support groups for people with hypertension. These groups focused on advice on healthy eating and exercise and, to a far lesser degree, on stress management. This woman was not hypertensive, but she joined the hypertension group, enjoyed it immensely, and gained a great deal of support from it. Her mood improved greatly. If we wished to label her behaviour, we might invoke hypotheses about somatization (see

Chapter 6), but this would be missing the point of her behaviour. She was an example of a person to whom the boundaries between 'mental health' and 'physical health' do not have the same meaning as for us, and she was able to find what she needed in an unexpected place. Ideally, our services should be such that people can cross our culturally constructed interdisciplinary boundaries and find help where it feels most appropriate to them. Our job, in working in an intersectoral way, is to anticipate that there may well be different interpretations, priorities, and aims across different disciplines. Once we can identify these differences, we are in a better position to find an appropriate place for our own contribution. In situations of poverty, in particular, it is often difficult to maintain a perspective which sees mental health as anything other than a luxury. Poverty, though, can lead to a cycle of demoralization which can seriously affect the quality of parent-infant interaction, for example, and we know that this interaction can have profound implications for subsequent development (Halpern, 1993). Breaking this cycle is a question not only of economics, but also of psychological change.

The term 'intersectoral collaboration' is generally used to refer to collaboration across different formal sectors such as health, education, welfare, and so on. It can, however, also be taken to refer to collaboration between professionals and the folk sector in mental health care, and in Africa much work has been done on collaboration with indigenous healers. In earlier chapters we have seen that use of multiple healing systems is the norm (Binitie, 1991). The Alma Ata conference (WHO,1978) saw indigenous or traditional healers as important resources in health care. Much is to be gained by a mutually respectful relationship between different healing sectors (Ben-Tovim, 1987). It is also, however, very important not to be romantic about what indigenous healing has to offer. A relationship of respect is not one of simply accepting that a system is effective without interrogating both its strengths and weaknesses, as we have seen throughout this book. Velimirovic (1990) launches a strident attack on what he terms the 'jumping on the bandwagon' of assuming that traditional medicine is always best for community well-being, without collecting evidence to support this view, and he argues against biases social scientists may hold 'toward cultural maintenance of diversity for its own sake' (Velimirovic, 1990: 72). If any claims are made that an approach is acceptable to a community or cultural group, and that it works, it should be possible to back these claims up by some evidence. What may be termed political correctness in terms of supporting diversity for its own sake is no substitute for trying to find out what helps people and what does not, and much damage can be done by romanticizing indigenous approaches (Farmer, 1997). There is also a difference between accepting that patients use a variety of services and assuming that, because of this, non-Western services are better than biomedicine. Much more work needs to be done which critically examines the interface between indigenous healing and professional mental health care, so that the best can be gained from both approaches, in the interests of the users of these services.

Cross-cultural interviewing and counselling

Many of the issues discussed thus far assume the collaborative work of people from various backgrounds, professional and/or personal. In a diverse society, though, there will always be direct clinical contacts between clinicians and clients from very different backgrounds. Many of the issues that pertain to work of this kind have been raised in the discussion of working with interpreters in Chapter 2. Even where the languages spoken by clinician and client are the same, cultural differences may well be a feature of the work. There are excellent training packages and approaches available to assist clinicians in cross-cultural counselling (Pedersen, in press; Ponterotto et al., 1995). A key factor in the field is how cultural issues intersect with issues of power, and the importance of being aware of political factors in this type of work cannot be stressed too strongly (Kareem & Littlewood, 1992).

Though interpersonal skills are undoubtedly important in intercultural interviews and therapy, it is at least as important to have a sense of what is happening in the interview room and why. Many of the lessons about interpreting and therapy and counselling apply here too. It may be a daunting task to try to establish a relationship with someone who feels very different from oneself. Not wishing to appear stupid or culturally insensitive can also be a great problem. This can lead to clinicians' pretending to understand when they do not. It is far better to ask directly about cultural beliefs (and possibly to look ignorant) than to conceal ignorance by not asking. This dishonesty, though understandable, must impact on the relationship with the client in a negative way. People are often grateful and relieved to be asked directly and respectfully about what they believe. At times, of course, people will use cultural difference as what has been termed 'cultural camouflage' (DiNicola, 1986). In other words, they will attempt to mask their problems or block access on the part of the clinician by claiming cultural difference as a basis for misunderstanding. Clinical skills are necessary to determine the degree to which cultural difference is being used in this way. If the clinician is reluctant to reveal less than perfect knowledge of the client's culture, *both* clinician and patient may end up being camouflaged by the illusion of impenetrable cultural differences. If people want to work together to solve a problem, on the other hand, they will generally find a way.

Until now, I have been speaking of intercultural therapy and counselling as though it occurs only between an individual client and an individual clinician. When I first started doing trauma work it was brought home to me how incorrect this view can be. I was asked to see a young man, about 18 years of age, to help him after he had been affected by political violence. Three generations appeared at my office with him – his siblings, his parents and aunt, and his grandmother. It has been suggested that some cultural groups are better suited to family or group therapy than to individual work (McGoldrick et al., 1982). Certainly, flexibility with respect to who attends counselling is useful, and great value can be gained from working with the people in the client's environment. Family therapy is, by its very nature, a more public activity than individual work, and may help people feel included in a process which otherwise may feel very foreign and strange to them. There is no evidence, though, that family or group work is automatically and inevitably better than other work – once again, it is important to think about what may be best in a given situation. Often the views of clients themselves may be very helpful in this regard.

Broader policy issues

How do we put what we know about culture and mental health to work in order to develop appropriate mental health policies? An important lesson from the literature on culture and mental health is that different people will view difficulties and challenges differently. A mental health system which makes no allowance for the range of interpretations which people have about health, illness, and well-being will not adequately meet people's needs. This means that some local participation in deciding on mental health priorities is necessary. Community participation in health and mental health issues is not always easy to achieve or evaluate, nor is it something which can replace careful thinking on the planners' part about what they would like to see happening in a community (Katzenellenbogen et al., 1997; Louw et al., 1995). Although there are obvious difficulties when professionals impose policies on communities, it is equally problematic when professionals hold back their views too much, as this may be withholding important professional knowledge which not everybody has access to. A situation of dialogue between different models and approaches is the ideal.

Given the fact that mental illness is stigmatized in different ways throughout the world (cf. Murphy, 1976), it is always important to anticipate that mental health issues may be very low on the agenda of communities and policy-making bodies. It is useful to remember that people with serious mental disorder and handicap are in many cases not allowed to vote in elections, so looking after them in a democracy is not of immediate vote-catching benefit for politicians. Part of our job is to look for ways to convince community leaders and politicians about the importance of mental health issues for the general good, both emotional and economic. This has been superbly done in the *World mental health* report (Desjarlais et al., 1995), which has suggested an agenda for action in the mental health area including the following points:

1 A major initiative to upgrade quality of mental heath services in Africa, Asia, Latin America, and the Middle East.
2 Upgrading of training in mental health for personnel at all levels, including medical students, graduate physicians, nurses and community health workers.
3 Empowerment of women economically, and reduction of violence against women, and the assessment of the broad mental health impact of such programmes.
4 Improvements in mental health services for children and adolescents, early detection and prevention of mental disorders, and educational programmes.
5 Concerted intervention in the area of prevention and treatment of substance (alcohol and drug) abuse.
6 Initiatives to attend to the causes and consequences of interpersonal violence.
7 A major focus on primary prevention of mental, neurological, behavioural, and psychosocial disorders. (Extracted from Desjarlais et al., 1995: 259-278)

The *World mental health* report plans are ambitious but necessary, and are especially convincing in that they relate mental health issues to much broader social concerns. This enables sectors other than the health or mental health sector to have a stake in the improvement of mental health world-wide.

The African launch of the *World mental health* report in Cape Town towards the end of 1995 coincided with a conference on mental health policy issues for South Africa. A volume on mental health policy issues for South Africa edited by, amongst others, the South African Director for Mental Health and Substance Abuse has recently appeared (Foster et al., 1997). Cultural factors were frequently mentioned at the conference, at which policy-makers from many other southern African countries were present, and it will be important to consider carefully the recommendations made in the volume in the light of a critical understanding of these factors (cf. Swartz, 1996).

The battle to give mental health issues the prominence they deserve, especially in Africa at this time, is of course a political battle (Dawes, 1986), but it is also a cultural one. We need to challenge relegation of mental health issues, and issues of the emotions more generally, to an arena commonly seen as less important than other concerns. In South Africa, the Truth and Reconciliation Commission (see Chapter 8) is playing an important role in bringing into sharp public focus the importance of mental health issues. The TRC has been likened to ancient Greek theatre, which brought hidden social and political concerns out into the open (Gevisser, 1997). Perhaps one of the lasting benefits of the Commission will be a greater public consciousness of the consequences of ignoring issues of human rights, human dignity, and the emotions in any society. South Africans in particular have an opportunity to put the visible issues of the damage of the apartheid years to building policies which consciously consider the importance of mental health outcomes.

The question of research

It is almost a ritual for academics to end off their books and articles with a call for more research. It is partly through such calls that we ensure our own professional life continues in a legitimate way! Given that more research is bound to happen, though, what can we learn from the issues raised in this book for mental health research in our region?

A fundamental issue is that no single approach will provide all the answers about any field. For example, the international quantitative research on serious mental disorder discussed in Chapter 9 produced important hypotheses which have been taken further and questioned by a more hermeneutic and critical approach. A range of research approaches are needed, and interdisciplinary research which facilitates the best work on the part of all participants is necessary (Swartz &

Miller, 1992b). A common and dangerous misconception about cultural studies of mental health issues is that they are in opposition to biological approaches. A culturally appropriate research agenda will be able to take the best from biological and social research, and to avoid extravagant and exclusive claims being made about any single approach.

Community participation in research, as in action programmes (Katzenellenbogen et al., 1997), is likely not only to provide information of local relevance, but also to teach researchers what the key cultural issues are in the particular research area. The question of culture in research is so loaded and politicized that researchers are often frightened to engage with it. In South Africa, for example, 'racial' categories are so strongly associated with appalling political oppression that some researchers are reluctant to identify their respondents in terms of 'race'. There are many instances, though, where knowing about a person's racial classification in terms of the apartheid categories is important. White people, for example, have had very different experiences of the health system in this country over the past century than have coloured people, who in turn have had different experiences from Africans, Indians, and so on. To make a statement such as this does not imply that I accept that the apartheid categories reflect cultural identities defined by people themselves. But the categories had profound consequences, including economic and emotional consequences. These consequences continue to be felt.

Intervention research is important – we need to test out the implementation of mental health programmes and to see what works, and what does not, as resources are scarce. Intervention studies, though, are not the only way we learn important information. Careful ethnographic accounts of mental health issues are relatively rare in our region, but such accounts can provide very useful information which will facilitate the culturally appropriate delivery of services. I am often struck by the amount of information people have about mental health issues but how there is often a reluctance to publish this information. Publishing requires confidence and certain skills; educators in particular have a responsibility to mentor others and to assist them to tell the world what they already know. There is a mystique about good research. Good research is not necessarily the most painful and difficult to do. If we respect local knowledge as part of our theoretical orientation, then we need to find ways to help this knowledge to be communicated and used for action.

The scope of mental health work

Where does mental health work begin and end? As we have seen throughout this book, the categories we use to divide the world into the 'mental' and the 'physical', into the realm of 'health' versus the arena of 'welfare', and so on, are cultural constructions. The concept of 'mental health' relies on a culturally specific medical view of human behaviour. A strong argument has been made, both internationally and locally, for expanding the focus of mental health interests to include broader social, economic, and political issues (Desjarlais et al., 1995; Petersen et al., 1996). There is no question that the expertise of mental health workers can contribute much to interventions outside the narrow area of mental disorders and their treatment and prevention. We also know that the overwhelming majority of mental health symptoms – chiefly anxiety and depression – will never come to the attention of mental health professionals. A broad approach seems an obvious one to take.

While it is true, though, that mental health is inseparable from all other aspects of well-being there are some dangers in being too all-inclusive. One of the consequences of the Alma Ata Declaration (WHO,1978), which had a very inclusive definition of health and health work, may be a tendency to feel overwhelmed by the extent of the task at hand. As we have seen, some CHW programmes have been shown to retreat into curative work with easily observable outcomes (Wood, 1990). It is also possible that by focusing too broadly, mental health workers may lose sight of the needs of stigmatized groups who have traditionally been their focus of interest – such as people with serious mental disorder and mental handicap. A balance is therefore needed between thinking broadly and retaining, at the very least, an advocacy function on behalf of those who, according to the cultural construction of the professions, have been designated as narrowly the responsibility of mental health workers.

Thinking about culture and mental health

This book is about ways of looking at the world and about ways of thinking about the world. I have argued throughout that there are always many ways of seeing things, and that these different approaches are often complementary. Understanding culture and mental health is not so much about knowing about a range of different experiences and practices as it is about having a way of trying to interpret what we see around us. There is nothing in the mental health field, anywhere in the world, professional, popular, or lay, which is not cultural. We all make meaning of our lives in the light of our own experiences and those of people around us.

The cultural challenge to mental health work is to move our usual practices, and those of everyone else, from the centre stage. No mental health practice is 'natural', and no group 'naturally' makes use of particular healing systems and approaches. These practices have all developed in historical contexts, and they are all changing all the time. A contemporary cultural approach to mental health issues recognizes diversity and recognizes change. The issues we face are not so much those of 'the X tribe do Y' type. They are instead questions about how people in a changing and interconnected world negotiate their lives and think and behave with respect to mental health issues, and more generally.

What I hope this book has given is not an encyclopaedia of different practices but instead examples of ways we can ask useful questions. If we can think about cultural issues in the mental health field, then we do not have to be frightened by new or changing information. The fact that the world is changing should represent for us exciting possibilities to develop our thinking further and, hence, to help people more effectively. Thinking culturally is all about reflection in the face of what the world offers us. It is about trying to make sense of what we see, and not about applying cultural labels to what we see. If we can allow ourselves to think and to ask questions, many positive effects will follow. The design and implementation of mental health programmes will be properly negotiated locally. The imposition of irrelevant and hurtful cultural labels will be avoided. Boundaries between groups of people begin to feel less absolute and terrifying if we can think and ask questions, not only about others but also about ourselves. The challenges we face are enormous. Thinking about them is one of our strongest tools.

references

Abas, M. A., & Broadhead, J. C.
1997   Depression and anxiety among women in an urban setting in Zimbabwe. *Psychological Medicine, 27*, 59–71.

Abas, M., Broadhead, J., Blue, I., Lewis, G., & Araya, R.
1995   Health service and community-based responses to mental ill-health in urban areas. In T. Harpham & I. Blue (Eds.). *Urbanization and mental health in developing countries* (pp. 227–248). Aldershot: Avebury.

Abas, M., Broadhead, J., Mbape, P., & Khumalo-Sakatukwa, G.
1994   Defeating depression in the developing world: A Zimbabwean model. *British Journal of Psychiatry, 164*, 293–296.

Abbott, A.
1988   *The system of the professions: An essay on the division of expert labor.* Chicago: University of Chicago Press.

Acharyya, S.
1992   The doctor's dilemma: The practice of cultural psychiatry in multicultural Britain. In J. Kareem & R. Littlewood (Eds.). *Intercultural therapy: Themes, interpretations and practice* (pp. 75–82). Oxford: Blackwell Scientific Publications.

Ainsworth, M.
1967   *Infancy in Uganda: Infant care and the growth of love.* Baltimore: Johns Hopkins University Press.

Akyeampong, E.
1995   Alcoholism in Ghana: A sociocultural exploration. *Culture, Medicine and Psychiatry, 19*, 261–280.

Almedom, A. M., & Abraham, S.
1994   Women, moral virtue and *tchat* chewing. In M. McDonald (Ed.). *Gender, drink and drugs* (pp. 249–259). Oxford: Berg Publishers.

American Psychiatric Association (APA)
1980   *Diagnostic and statistical manual of mental disorders* (3rd ed.) (DSM-III). Washington, D.C.: American Psychiatric Association.
1987   *Diagnostic and statistical manual of mental disorders* (3rd ed., revised)

(DSM-III-R). Washington, D.C.: American Psychiatric Association.

1994   *Diagnostic and statistical manual of mental disorders* (4th ed.) (DSM-IV). Washington, D.C.: American Psychiatric Association.

Andersson, N., & Marks, S.

1988   Apartheid and health in the 1980s. *Social Science and Medicine*, **27**, 667–682.

Anonymous

1986   Some thoughts on a more relevant or indigenous counselling psychology in South Africa. *Psychology in Society*, **5**, 81–89.

Arluke, A.

1980   Roundsmanship: Inherent control on a medical teaching ward. *Social Science and Medicine*, **14A**, 297–302.

Armstrong, D.

1987   Theoretical tensions in biopsychosocial medicine. *Social Science and Medicine*, **25**, 1213–1218.

Asuni, T.

1967   Tropical neuropathy and psychosis. *British Journal of Psychiatry*, **113**, 1031–1033.

Asuni, T. S.

1991   Development of psychiatry in Africa. In S. O. Okpaku (Ed.). *Mental health in Africa and the Americas today* (pp. 17-32). Nashville: Crisolith Books.

Asuni, T., Schoenberg, F., & Swift, C.

1994   *Mental health and disease in Africa*. Ibadan: Spectrum Books Limited.

Ball, A., & Howard, J.

1995   Psychoactive substance abuse among street children. In T. Harpham & I. Blue (Eds.). *Urbanization and mental health in developing countries* (pp. 123–149). Aldershot: Avebury.

Barker, P.

1991   *Regeneration*. Harmondsworth: Penguin.

1993   *The eye at the door*. Harmondsworth: Penguin.

1995   *The ghost road*. Harmondsworth: Penguin.

Barrelet, L., Ferrero, F., Szigethy, L., Giddey, C., & Pellizzer, G.

1990   Expressed emotion and first-admission schizophrenia: Nine-month follow-up in a French cultural environment. *British Journal of Psychiatry*, **156**, 357–362.

Barrett, R.

1996   *The psychiatric team and the social definition of schizophrenia: An anthropological study of person and illness*. Cambridge: Cambridge University Press.

Barrett, R. J.
1988   Clinical writing and the documentary construction of schizophrenia.
         Culture, Medicine and Psychiatry, **12**, 265–299.

Bass, N.
1996   *A qualitative exploration of the UCT Child Guidance Clinic's bicultural
         workers programme: Can formalised mentoring programmes assist in the
         transformation of South African Clinical Psychology?* Unpublished psychology
         honours research project, University of Cape Town.

Beaglehole, R., Bonita, R., & Kjellström, T.
1993   *Basic epidemiology.* Geneva: World Health Organization.

Beck, A. T., Rush, A. J., Shaw, B. F., & Emery, G. (Eds.)
1979   *Cognitive therapy of depression.* New York: Guilford Press.

Becker, D., Lira, E., Castillo, M., Gomez, E., & Kovalskys, J.
1995   Therapy with victims of political repression in Chile: The challenge of
         social reparation. In N. J. Kritz (Ed.). *Transitional justice: How emerging
         democracies reckon with former regimes. Volume 1: General considerations*
         (pp. 583–591). Washington, D.C.: United States Institute of Peace Press.

Belli, R. F., & Loftus, E. F.
1994   Recovered memories of childhood abuse: A source monitoring perspective.
         In S. J. Lynn & J. W. Rhue (Eds.). *Dissociation: Clinical and theoretical
         perspectives* (pp. 415–433). New York: Guilford Press.

Ben-Arie, O., Swartz, L., & Dickman, B. J.
1987   Depression in the elderly living in the community: Its presentation and
         features. *British Journal of Psychiatry*, **150**, 169–174.

Ben-Tovim, D.
1987   *Development psychiatry: Mental health and primary health care in Botswana.*
         London: Tavistock.

Berger, S., & Lazarus, S.
1987   The views of community organisers on the relevance of psychological
         practice in South Africa. *Psychology in Society*, 7, 6–23.

Berry, J. W.
1995   Psychology of acculturation. In N. R. Goldberger & J. B. Veroff (Eds.).
         The culture and psychology reader (pp. 457–488). New York: New York
         University Press.

Berry, J. W., & Kim, U.
1993   The way ahead: From indigenous psychologies to a universal psychology.
         In U. Kim & J. W. Berry (Eds.). *Indigenous psychologies: Research experience in
         cultural context* (pp. 260–280). Newbury Park: Sage.

Beusenberg, M., & Orley, J.
1994   *A user's guide to the Self-Reporting Questionnaire.* Geneva: World Health
        Organization.

Bevis, W. M.
1921   Psychological traits of the Southern Negro with observations as to some of
        his psychoses. *American Journal of Psychiatry,* **1**, 69–78.

Bibeau, G.
1997   Cultural psychiatry in a creolizing world: Questions for a new research
        agenda. *Transcultural Psychiatry,* **34**, 9–41.

Biko, S.
1978   *I write what I like.* London: Bowerdean Press.

Binedell, J.
1991   Community health workers talk about their work. Presented at the
        Association for Sociology of Southern Africa conference, University of
        Cape Town, July.
1993   *Methods and madness: Researching community health workers' perceptions of
        mental illness in Khayelitsha and Nyanga.* Unpublished M.A. thesis,
        University of Cape Town.

Binitie, A.
1971   *A study of depression in Benin Nigeria.* Unpublished Ph.D. dissertation,
        University of London.
1991   The mentally ill in modern and traditional African societies. In S. O.
        Okpaku (Ed.). *Mental health in Africa and the Americas today* (pp. 1–15).
        Nashville: Crisolith Books.

Blouin, J., Spindler, E., Perez, E., Blouin, A., Hotz, S., & Hakkaku, J.
1992   The role of stress in interpreting the dexamethasone suppression test.
        Canadian Journal of Psychiatry, **37**, 724–727.

Blue, I., & Harpham, T.
1994   The World Bank *World development report 1993: Investing in health*:
        Reveals the burden of common mental disorders, but ignores its
        implications. *British Journal of Psychiatry,* **165**, 9–12.

Blumberg, J., Swartz, L., & Roper, K.
1996   Possibilities for intervention in wife abuse: Discourses among care givers in
        a community health project. In L. Glanz & A. D. Spiegel (Eds.). *Violence and
        family life in contemporary South Africa: Research and policy issues*
        (pp. 167–200). Pretoria: HSRC.

Blumhagen, D.
1980   Hyper-tension: A folk illness with a medical name. *Culture, Medicine and
        Psychiatry,* **4**, 197–213.

1982   The meaning of hyper-tension. In N. J. Chrisman & T. W. Maretzki (Eds.). *Clinically applied anthropology* (pp. 297–323). Dordrecht: Reidel.

Boonzaier, E.

1985   Choice of healer: An important area of interest for general practitioners. *South African Family Practice*, **6**, 235–240.

Boonzaier, E., & Sharp, J. (Eds.)

1988   *South African keywords: The use and abuse of political concepts.* Cape Town: David Philip.

Breslau, N., Davis, C. G., Peterson, E. L., & Schultz, L.

1997   Psychiatric sequelae of posttraumatic stress in women. *Archives of General Psychiatry*, **54**, 81–87.

Brislin, R. W.

1986   The wording and translation of research instruments. In W. J. Lonner & J. W. Berry (Eds.). *Field-methods in cross-cultural research* (pp. 137–164). Berkeley: Sage Publications.

Brittain, V., & Minty, A. S. (Eds.)

1988   *Children of resistance: On children, repression and the law in apartheid South Africa (Statements from the Harare conference).* London: Kliptown.

Brown, G. L., Albaugh, B. J., Robin, R. W., Goodson, S. G., Trunzo, M., Wynne, D. K., & Goldman, D.

1993   Alcoholism and substance abuse among selected Southern Cheyenne Indians. *Culture, Medicine and Psychiatry*, **16**, 531–542.

Brown, G. W., Birley, J. L. T., & Wing, J. K.

1972   Influence of family life on the course of schizophrenic disorders: A replication. *British Journal of Psychiatry*, **121**, 241–258.

Bührmann, M. V.

1977   Western psychiatry and the Xhosa patient. *South African Medical Journal*, **51**, 464–466.

1981   The Xhosa healers of Southern Africa. 1. Intlombe and xhentsa: A Xhosa healing ritual. *Journal of Analytical Psychology*, **26**, 187–201.

1982   Thwasa and bewitchment. *South African Medical Journal*, **61**, 877–879.

1983a   Archetypal transference as observed in the healing procedures of Xhosa amagqira. In J. Beebe (Ed.). *Money, food, drink and fashion and analytical training: Depth dimensions of physical existence.* (Papers of the 8th International Congress of Analytical Psychology) (pp. 249–258). Fellbach-Oeffingen (W. Germany): Bonz.

1983b   Training of Xhosa medicine-men and analytical psychologists: A comparative study. In J. Beebe (Ed.). *Money, food, drink and fashion and analytical training: Depth dimensions of physical existence.* (Papers of the 8th International Congress of Analytical Psychology) (pp. 237–245). Fellbach-Oeffingen (W. Germany): Bonz.

1984   *Living in two worlds: Communication between a white healer and her black counterparts*. Cape Town: Human & Rousseau.

Bührmann, M. V., & Gqomfa, J. N.

1981   The Xhosa healers of Southern Africa. 2. The songs sung in a healing ceremony. *Journal of Analytical Psychology, 26*, 297–312.

1982a   The Xhosa healers of Southern Africa. 3. A family therapy session with a dream as central content. *Journal of Analytical Psychology, 27*, 41–57.

1982b   The Xhosa healers of Southern Africa. 4. Isiko lentambo: A renewal sacrifice. *Journal of Analytical Psychology, 27*, 163–173.

Butchart, R. A.

1996   *On the anatomy of power: Bodies of knowledge in South African socio-medical discourse*. Unpublished D. Litt. et Phil. dissertation, University of South Africa, Pretoria.

Carter, R. T., & Qureshi, A.

1995   A typology of philosophical assumptions in multicultural counseling and training. In J. G. Ponterotto, J. M. Casas, L. A. Suzuki, & C. M. Alexander (Eds.). *Handbook of multicultural counseling* (pp. 237–262). Thousand Oaks, California: Sage.

Cassidy, C. M.

1982   Protein-energy malnutrition as a culture-bound syndrome. *Culture, Medicine and Psychiatry, 6*, 325–345.

Castillo, R. J.

1994a   Spirit possession in South Asia, dissociation or hysteria? Part 1: Theoretical background. *Culture, Medicine and Psychiatry, 18*, 1–21.

1994b   Spirit possession in South Asia, dissociation or hysteria? Part 2: Case histories. *Culture, Medicine and Psychiatry, 18*, 141–162.

1997   *Culture and mental illness: A client-centered approach*. Pacific Grove, California: Brooks/Cole.

Centre for the Study of Health Policy

1990   *The need for improved mental health care in South Africa*. Briefing Document, Centre for the Study of Health Policy, University of the Witwatersrand, Johannesburg.

Chavunduka, G.

1994   *Traditional medicine in modern Zimbabwe*. Harare: University of Zimbabwe Publications.

Cheetham, R. W. S., & Griffiths, J. A.

1982   Sickness and medicine — an African paradigm. *South African Medical Journal, 62*, 954–956.

Claridge, G.

1970   *Drugs and human behaviour*. London: Allen Lane.

Clifford, J.
1986   *Writing culture: The poetics and politics of ethnography.* Berkeley: University of California Press.

Cohen, A.
1992   Prognosis for schizophrenia in the Third World: A reevaluation of cross-cultural research. *Culture, Medicine and Psychiatry,* **16**, 53–75.

Collins, P. Y., Wig, N. N., Day, R., Varma, V. K., Malhorta, S., Misra, A. K., Schanzer, B., & Susser, E.
1996   Psychosocial and biological aspects of acute brief psychoses in developing country sites. *Psychiatric Quarterly,* **67** (3), 177–193.

Comaroff, J.
1985   *Body of power, spirit of resistance. The culture and history of a South African people.* Chicago: University of Chicago Press.

Committee to Study Female Morbidity and Mortality in Sub-Saharan Africa
1996   Mental health problems. In C. P. Howson, P. F. Harrison., D. Hotra, & M. Law (Eds.). *In her lifetime: Female morbidity and mortality in sub-Saharan Africa* (pp. 136–151). Washington, D.C.: National Academy Press. Note: In the introduction to the volume, J. Orley and and G. De Girolamo are cited as 'primary authors' of the chapter.

Committee to Visit South Africa (Stone, A., Pinder-Hughes, C., Spurlock, J., & Weinberg, D.)
1979   Report of the Committee to Visit South Africa. *American Journal of Psychiatry,* **136**, 1498–1506.

Cooper, J. E., Kendell, R. E., Gurland, B. J., Sharpe, L., Copeland, J. R. M., & Simon, R.
1972   *Psychiatric diagnosis in New York and London.*London: Oxford University Press.

Craig, T. J., Siegel, C., Hopper, K., Lin, S., & Sartorius, N.
1997   Outcome in schizophrenia and related disorders compared between developing and developed countries: A recursive partitioning re-analysis of the WHO DOSMD data. *British Journal of Psychiatry,* **170**, 229–233.

Crawford, A.
1994   *Black patients/white doctors: Stories lost in translation.* Cape Town: National Language Project.

Csordas, T. J.
1994   *The sacred self: A cultural phenomenology of charismatic healing.* Berkeley: University of California Press.

Dasen, P. R., Berry, J. W., & Sartorius, N. (Eds.)
1988   *Health and cross-cultural psychology: Towards applications.* Newbury Park: Sage.

Davis, D. L.
1989a   George Beard and Lydia Pinkham: Gender, class, and nerves in late 19th
         century America. In D. L. Davis & S. M. Low (Eds.). *Gender, health and
         illness: The case of nerves* (pp. 1–22). New York: Hemisphere Publishing
         Corporation.
1989b   The variable character of nerves in a Newfoundland fishing village.
         Medical Anthropology, **11**, 63–78.

Davis, D. L., & Guarnaccia, P. J.
1989   Health, culture and the nature of nerves; Introduction. *Medical Anthropology*,
        11, 1–13.

Davis, D. L., & Low, S. M. (Eds.)
1989   *Gender, health and illness: The case of nerves*. New York: Hemisphere
        Publishing Corporation.

Davis, D. L., & Whitten, R. G.
1988   Medical and popular traditions of nerves. *Social Science and Medicine*,
        26, 1209–1221.

Dawes, A. R. L.
1985   Politics and mental health: The position of clinical psychology in South
        Africa. *South African Journal of Psychology* **15**, 55–61.
1986   The notion of relevant psychology with particular reference to Africanist
        pragmatic initiatives. *Psychology in Society*, **5**, 28–48.

Dawes, A. R. L., & De Villiers, C.
1989   Preparing children and their parents for prison: The Wynberg 7. In J. B.
        Mason & J. Rubenstein (Eds.). *Family therapy in South Africa today*
        (pp. 15–23). Congella, South Africa: South African Institute of Marital
        and Family Therapy.

Dawes, A. R. L., Tredoux, C., & Feinstein, A.
1989   Political violence in South Africa: Some effects on children of the violent
        destruction of their community. *International Journal of Mental Health*,
        18 (2), 16–43.

Daynes, G., & Msengi, N. P.
1979   'Why am I ill? Who made me ill?' The relevance of Western psychiatry in
        Transkei. *South African Medical Journal*, **56**, 307–310.

De Beer, C.
1986   Apartheid, health and health services in South Africa. Proceedings of the
        Organization for Appropriate Social Services in Southern Africa 'Apartheid
        and Mental Health' Conference (pp. 13–20). Johannesburg: OASSSA.

De Jesus Mari, J., & Streiner, D. L.
1994   An overview of family interventions and relapse in schizophrenia:
        Meta-analysis of research findings. *Psychological Medicine*, **24**, 565–578.

Desjarlais, R., Eisenberg, L., Good, B., & Kleinman, A.
1995   *World mental health: Problems and priorities in low-income countries.*
        New York and Oxford: Oxford University Press.

Dhadphale, M., & Ellison, R. H.
1983   The frequency of mental disorders in the outpatients of two Nyanza
        hospitals. *The Central African Journal of Medicine,* **29,** 29–32.

Dinges, N. G., & Duong-Tran, Q.
1993   Stressful life events and co-occurring depression, substance abuse and
        suicidality among American Indian and Alaska Native adolescents.
        Culture, Medicine and Psychiatry, **16,** 487–502.

DiNicola, V. F.
1986   Beyond Babel: Family therapy as cultural transition. *International Journal*
        of Family Therapy, 7, 179–191.
1990   Anorexia multiforme: Self-starvation in historical and cultural context, II.
        Anorexia nervosa as a culture-reactive syndrome.*Transcultural Psychiatric*
        Research Review, **27,** 245–286.

Dixon, J. A.
1997   Discourse and racial partition in the 'new' South Africa. In A. Levett, A.
        Kottler, E. Burman, & I. Parker (Eds.). *Culture, power and difference:*
        Discourse analysis in South Africa (pp. 17–30). London: Zed Books, and
        Cape Town: University of Cape Town Press.

Dixon, J. A., Foster, D. H., Durrheim, K., & Wilbraham, L.
1994   Discourse and the politics of space in South Africa: The 'squatter crisis'.
        Discourse and Society, **5,** 277–296.

Dommisse, J.
1984a   Apartheid as a public mental health issue. Paper presented at the World
        Psychiatric Association Regional Symposium, Helsinki, June.
1984b   The psychological effects of apartheid (South African Naziism). Paper
        presented to the American Academy of Psychoanalysis 28th Winter
        Meeting, New York, December.
1986   The state of psychiatry in South Africa today (1986). Paper presented at the
        Third African National Congress Health Council, Lusaka, June.
1987   The state of psychiatry in South Africa today. *Social Science and Medicine,*
        24, 749–761 (includes comments by S. D. Edwards and by S. P. Sashidharan
        & S. Platt, referenced separately, and a rejoinder by Dommisse).

Doyal, L.
1995   *What makes women sick: Gender and the political economy of health.*
        London: Macmillan.

Drennan, G.
1996a   Counting the cost of language services in psychiatry. *South African*
        Medical Journal, **86,** 343–345.

1996b   Institutional obstacles to equitable access to psychiatric services in the
         Western Cape. Paper presented at the conference: Communication for the
         health professional in a multi-lingual society, University of Natal, Durban,
         11 July 1996.

in press Psychiatry, post-apartheid integration and the neglected role of language
          in South African institutional contexts. *Transcultural Psychiatry.*

Drennan, G., Levett, A., & Swartz, L.
1991   Hidden dimensions of power and resistance in the translation process:
          A South African study. *Culture, Medicine and Psychiatry*, **15**, 361–381.

DSM-III
1980   *See* American Psychiatric Association.

DSM-III-R
1987   *See* American Psychiatric Association.

DSM-IV
1994   *See* American Psychiatric Association.

Dunk, P.
1989   Greek women and broken nerves in Montreal. *Medical Anthropology*,
          11, 29–45.

Ebigbo, P.
1982   Development of a cultural specific screening scale for somatic complaints
          indicating psychiatric disturbance. *Culture, Medicine and Psychiatry*, **6**, 29–43.

Edgerton, R., & Cohen, A.
1994   Culture and schizophrenia: The DOSMD challenge. *British Journal of
          Psychiatry*, **164**, 222–231.

Edwards, F. S.
1983a   Amafufunyana spirit possession: A report on some current developments.
          Paper presented at the Fifth Annual Congress for the Study of Religion.
          University of Durban-Westville, June/July.
1983b   Healing and transculturation in Xhosa Zionist practice. *Culture, Medicine
          and Psychiatry*, **7**, 177–198.

Edwards, S. D.
1986   Traditional and modern medicine in South Africa: A research study.
          Social Science and Medicine, **22**, 1273–1276.
1987   Comment on 'The state of psychiatry in South Africa today' by John
          Dommisse. *Social Science and Medicine*, **24**, 758.

Edwards, S. D., Cheetham, R. W. S., Majozi, E., & Lasisch, A.
1982   Zulu culture-bound psychiatric syndromes. *South African Journal of
          Hospital Medicine*, **8**, 82–86.

Eisenberg, L.

1986   Is there too much science in medicine or not enough? A position paper.
In S. McHugh & T. M. Vallis (Eds.). *Illness behaviour: A multidisciplinary model* (pp. 33–45). New York: Plenum Press.

1988   The social construction of mental illness. *Psychological Medicine*, **18**, 1–19.

1995   The social construction of the human brain. *American Journal of Psychiatry*, **152**, 1563–1575.

1996   Foreword. In J. E. Mezzich, A. Kleinman, H. Fabrega, Jr., & D. L. Parron, (Eds.). *Culture and diagnosis: A DSM-IV perspective* (pp. xiii-xv). Washington, D.C.: American Psychiatric Press.

Elk, R., Dickman, B. J., & Teggin, A. F.

1986   Depression in schizophrenia: A study of prevalence and treatment.
British Journal of Psychiatry, **149**, 228–229.

Engel, G.L.

1977   The need for a new medical model: A challenge for biomedicine.
Science, **196**, 129–136.

Ensink, K., & Robertson, B.

1996   Indigenous categories of distress and dysfunction in South African Xhosa children and adolescents as described by indigenous healers. *Transcultural Psychiatric Research Review*, **33**, 137–172.

1997   Patient and family experiences of psychiatric services and African indigenous healers. Unpublished paper, Department of Psychiatry, University of Cape Town.

Ensink, K., Roberston, B. A., Ben-Arie, O., Hodson, P., & Tredoux, C.

1997   Expression of schizophrenia in African Xhosa-speaking and white English-speaking South Africans. Unpublished paper, Department of Psychiatry, University of Cape Town.

Ensink, K., Roberston, B., Zissis, C., & Leger, P.

1997   Posttraumatic stress disorder in children exposed to violence. Unpublished paper, Department of Psychiatry, University of Cape Town.

Estroff, S.

1981   *Making it crazy: An ethnography of psychiatric clients in an American community.* Berkeley: University of California Press.

Fabrega, H.

1992   Biomedical psychiatry as an object for a critical medical anthropology.
In S. Lindenbaum & M. Lock (Eds.). *Knowledge, power and practice: The anthropology of medicine and everyday life.* Berkeley: University of California Press.

Fainzang, S.
1996   Alcoholism, a contagious disease. A contribution towards an anthropological definition of contagion. *Culture, Medicine and Psychiatry*, **20**, 473–487.

Fanon, F.
1970   *Black skin, white masks.* London: Paladin.

Farmer, P.
1996   On suffering and structural violence: A view from below. *Daedalus*, **125** (1), 261–283.
1997   Social scientists and the new tuberculosis. *Social Science and Medicine*, **44**, 347–358.

Farrand, D.
1980   *An analysis of indigenous healing in suburban Johannesburg.* Unpublished master's thesis, University of the Witwatersrand, Johannesburg.

Feierman, S., & Janzen, J. M. (Eds.)
1992   *The social basis of health and healing in Africa.* Berkeley: University of California Press.

Fernando, S.
1991   *Mental health, race, and culture.* London: Macmillan.

Finkler, K.
1989   The universality of nerves. In D. L. Davis & S. M. Low (Eds.). *Gender, health and illness: The case of nerves* (pp. 79–101). New York: Hemisphere Publishing Corporation.
1991   *Physicians at work, patients in pain: Biomedical practice and patient response in Mexico.* Boulder, Colorado: Westview Press.
1994   *Women in pain: Gender and morbidity in Mexico.* Philadelphia: University of Pennsylvania Press.

Fleming, C.
1996   Cultural formulation of psychiatric diagnosis. Case No 01: An American Indian woman suffering from depression, alcoholism and childhood trauma. *Culture, Medicine and Psychiatry*, **20**, 145–154.

Flisher, A. J., Ziervogel, C. F., Chalton, D. O., Leger, P. H., & Robertson, B. A.
1993a   Risk taking behaviour of Cape Peninsula high school students: IV. Alcohol use. *South African Medical Journal*, **83**, 480–482.
1993b   Risk taking behaviour of Cape Peninsula high school students: V. Drug use. *South African Medical Journal*, **83**, 483–485.

Foster, D., Davis, D., & Sandler, D.
1987   *Detention and torture in South Africa.* Cape Town: David Philip.

Foster, D., Freeman, M., & Pillay, Y. (Eds.)
1997   *Mental health policy issues for South Africa.* Cape Town: MASA Multimedia.

Foucault, M.

1973a   *Madness and civilization*. New York: Vintage.

1973b   *The birth of the clinic: An archaeology of medical perception*. New York: Vintage.

1979   *Discipline and punish: The birth of the prison*. New York: Vintage.

Frader, J. E., & Bosk, C.

1981   Parent talk at intensive care rounds. *Social Science and Medicine*, **15E**, 267–274.

Freed, E. D., & Bishop, E.

1980   Major psychiatric disability in open ward patients referred by medical and surgical units at Baragwanath Hospital: A study of 1889 patients. *The Leech*, **50** (3), 56–62.

Freeman, M.

1989   *Mental health care in crisis in South Africa*. Paper no.16, Centre for the Study of Health Policy, University of the Witwatersrand, Johannesburg.

1992   *Providing mental health care for all in South Africa: Structure and strategy*. Paper no. 24, Centre for Health Policy, University of the Witwatersrand, Johannesburg.

Freud, S.

1991/1905   *On sexuality: Three essays on sexuality and other works* (J. Strachey, Trans., A. Richards, Ed.). Harmondsworth: Penguin.

Gabe, J., Kelleher, D., & Williams, G. (Eds.)

1994   *Challenging medicine*. London and New York: Routledge.

Gater, R., De Almeida e Sousa, B., Barrientos, G., Caraveo, J., Chandrashekar, C. R., Dhadphale, M., Goldberg, D., Al Kathiri, A. H., Mubbashar, M., Silhan, K., Thong, D., Torres-Gonzales, F., & Sartorius, N.

1991   The pathways to psychiatric care: A cross-cultural study. *Psychological Medicine*, 21, 761–774.

Gevisser, M.

1997   The Mark Gevisser page. *The Sunday Independent*, 10 August.

Gifford, S. M.

1986   The meaning of lumps: A case study in the ambiguities of risk. In C. R. Janes, R. Stall, & S. M. Gifford (Eds.). *Anthropology and epidemiology* (pp. 213–246). Dordrecht: Reidel.

Gijana, E. W. M., & Louw, J.

1981   Psychiatric disorders in a developing community as reflected by archival material. *South African Medical Journal*, **59**, 988–991.

Gilbert, N., & Mulkay, M.

1984   *Opening Pandora's box: A sociological analysis of scientists' discourse*. Cambridge: Cambridge University Press.

Gillis, L. S.
1986a   *Guidelines in psychiatry* (3rd ed.). Cape Town: David Philip.
1986b   Readmissions to psychiatric hospitals (Editorial). *South African Medical Journal*, **70**, 715–716.
1987   Psychiatric research — a new tomorrow. *South African Medical Journal*, **72**, 797–799.
1992   Depression in newly-urbanised elderly South Africans. *Southern African Journal of Gerontology*, **1**, 20–24.

Gillis, L. S., Elk, R., Ben-Arie, O., & Teggin, A. F.
1982   The Present State Examination: Experiences with Xhosa-speaking psychiatric patients. *British Journal of Psychiatry*, **141**, 143–147.

Gillis, L. S., Jakoet, A., Trollip, D., Sandler, R., & Elk, R.
1987   The outcome of psychiatric illness: A two-year follow-up study. *South African Medical Journal*, **72**, 598–602.

Gillis, L. S., Koch, A., & Joyi, M.
1989   Improving compliance in Xhosa psychiatric patients. *South African Medical Journal*, **72**, 205–208.

Gillis, L. S., Sandler, R., Jakoet, A., & Elk, R.
1986a   Admissions to a psychiatric hospital: Factors associated with admission and inpatient care. *South African Medical Journal*, **70**, 731–734.
1986b   Readmissions to a psychiatric hospital: Outcome on follow-up. *South African Medical Journal*, **70**, 735–739.

Gillis, L. S., & Stone, G.L.
1973   A follow-up study of psychiatric disturbance in a Cape Coloured community. *British Journal of Psychiatry*, **123**, 279–283.

Gillis, L. S., Trollip, D., Jakoet, A., & Holden, T.
1987   Non-compliance with psychotropic medication. *South African Medical Journal*, **72**, 602–606.

Gilman, S. L.
1995   *Health and illness: Images of difference.* London: Reaktion Books.

Glass, J. M.
1993   *Shattered selves: Multiple personality in a postmodern world.* Ithaca and London: Cornell University Press.

Goffman, E.
1961   *Asylums.* New York: Doubleday.

Goldberg, D.
1978   *Manual of the General Health Questionnaire.* NFER Publishing: England.

Goldberg, D. P.
1972   *The detection of psychiatric illness by questionnaire* (Maudsley Monograph No. 21). London: Oxford University Press.

Goldberg, D. P., & Hillier, V. F.
1979   A scaled version of the General Health Questionnaire. *Psychological Medicine*, **9**, 139–145.

Goldberg, D., & Huxley, P.
1980   *Mental illness in the community.* London: Tavistock.
1992   *Common mental disorders: A bio-social model.* London: Routledge.

Good, B. J.
1977   The heart of what's the matter: The semantics of illness in Iran. *Culture, Medicine and Psychiatry*, **1**, 25–58.
1996   Culture and DSM-IV: Diagnosis, knowledge and power. *Culture, Medicine and Psychiatry*, **20**, 127–132.

Good, B. J., & Good, M.-J. DelVecchio
1980   The meaning of symptoms: A cultural hermeneutic model for clinical practice. In L. Eisenberg & A. Kleinman (Eds.). *The relevance of social science for medicine* (pp. 165–196). Dordrecht: Reidel.

Good, M.-J. DelVecchio, Brodwin, P., Good, B., & Kleinman, A. (Eds.)
1992   *Pain as human experience: An anthropological perspective.* Berkeley: University of California Press.

Gordon, D. R.
1988   Tenacious assumptions in western medicine. In M. Lock & D. Gordon (Eds.). *Biomedicine examined* (pp. 19–56). Dordrecht: Kluwer.

Green, E.C.
1997   Purity, pollution and the invisible snake in southern Africa. *Medical Anthropology*, **17**, 83–100.

Guarnaccia, P. J., DeLaCancela, V., & Carrillo, E.
1989   The multiple meanings of ataques de nervios in the Latino community. *Medical Anthropology*, **11**, 47–62.

Guarnaccia, P. J., & Farias, P.
1988   The social meanings of *nervios*: A case study of a Central American woman. *Social Science and Medicine*, **26**, 1223–1231.

Guarnaccia, P. J., Rubio-Stipec, M., & Canino, G.
1989   Ataques de nervios in the Puerto Rican diagnostic interview schedule: The impact of cultural categories on psychiatric epidemiology. *Culture, Medicine and Psychiatry*, **13**, 275–295.

Gureje, O., Mavreas, V., Vazquez-Barquero, J. L., & Janca, A.
1997   Problems related to alcohol use: A cross cultural perspective. *Culture, Medicine and Psychiatry*, **21**, 213–246.

Hacking, I.
1995   *Rewriting the soul: Multiple personality and the sciences of memory.* Princeton: Princeton University Press.

Hahn, R. A., & Gaines, A. D. (Eds.)
1985   *Physicians of western medicine: Anthropological approaches to theory and practice.* Dodrecht: Reidel.

Haley, J.
1976   *Problem-solving therapy: New strategies for effective family therapy.* New York: Harper Colophon Books.

Halpern, R.
1993   Poverty and infant development. In C. H. Zeanah, Jr. (Ed.). *Handbook of infant mental health* (pp. 73–86). New York: Guilford Press.

Hammond-Tooke, W. D.
1975   African world-view and its relevance for psychiatry. *Psychologia Africana,* **16**, 25–32.

Harding, T. W., De Arango, M. V., Baltazar, J., Climent, C. E., Ibrahim, H. H. A., Ladrido-Ignacio, L., Srinivasa Murthy, R., & Wig, N. N.
1980   Mental disorders in primary health care: A study of their frequency and diagnosis in four developing countries. *Psychological Medicine,* **17**, 231–241.

Harpham, T., & Blue, I. (Eds.)
1995   *Urbanization and mental health in developing countries.* Aldershot: Avebury.

Harpham, T., & Tanner, I. (Eds.)
1995   *Urban health in developing countries: Progress and prospects.* New York: St. Martin's Press.

Heap, M.
1986   A profile of a sample of Crossroads households and some survival strategies. Paper presented at the Western Cape Roots and Realities conference, Centre for African Studies, University of Cape Town, July.

Heller, K., Price, R. H., Reinharz, S., Riger, S., Wandersman, A., & D'Aunno, T. A. (Eds.)
1984   *Psychology and community change: Challenges of the future.* Pacific Grove, California: Brooks Cole.

Helman, C.
1987   Heart disease and the cultural construction of time: The Type A behaviour pattern as a western culture-bound syndrome. *Social Science and Medicine,* **25**, 969–979.
1991   *Body myths.* London: Chatto and Windus.
1994   *Culture, health and illness: An introduction for health professionals* (3rd ed.). Oxford: Butterworth-Heinemann.

Henriques, J., Hollway, W., Urwin, C., & Walkerdine, V.
1984   *Changing the subject. Psychology, social regulation and subjectivity.* London: Methuen.

Hickie, I., Lloyd, A., Hadzi-Pavlovic, D., Parker, G., & Wakefield, D.

1995   Can the chronic fatigue syndrome be defined by distinct clinical features?
         Psychological Medicine, **25**, 925–935.

Hirschowitz, R., & Orkin, M. (with J. De Castro, S. Hirschowitz, K. Segel,
& L Taunyane)

1995   *A national household survey of health inequalities in South Africa.*
         (Community Agency for Social Enquiry — CASE — survey for the Henry J.
         Kaiser Family Foundation.) Washington, D.C.: Henry J. Kaiser Family
         Foundation.

Hoffman, E.

1989   *Lost in translation: A life in a new language.* New York: E. P. Dutton.

Hoffman, M., Pick, W., Joubert, G., Yach, D., Thomas, T., & Klopper, J. M. L.

1988   Morbidity profile of the Mamre community. *South African Medical
         Journal*, **74**, 358–361.

Holdstock, T. L.

1981a   Indigenous healing in South Africa and the person-centered approach of
         Carl Rogers. *Curare*, **4**, 31–46.

1981b   Psychology in South Africa belongs to the colonial era: Arrogance or
         ignorance? *South African Journal of Psychology*, **11**, 123–129.

Hopper, K.

1991   Some old questions for the new cross-cultural psychiatry. *Medical
         Anthropology Quarterly*, **5**, 299–329.

1992   Cervantes' puzzle — a commentary on Alex Cohen's 'Prognosis for
         schizophrenia in the Third World: A reevaluation of cross-cultural
         research'. *Culture, Medicine and Psychiatry*, **16**, 89–100.

Howitt, D., & Owusu-Bempah, J.

1994   *The racism of psychology: Time for a change.* Hemel Hempstead:
         Harvester Wheatsheaf.

Howland, R. H., & Thase, M. E.

1991   Biological studies of dysthymia. *Biological Psychiatry*, **30**, 283–304.

Hughes, C. C.

1990   Ethnopsychiatry. In T. M. Johnson & C. E. Sargent (Eds.). *Medical
         anthropology: Contemporary theory and method* (pp. 132–148). New York:
         Praeger.

1996   The culture-bound syndromes and psychiatric diagnosis. In J. E. Mezzich,
         A.Kleinman, H. Fabrega, Jr., & D. L. Parron (Eds.). *Culture and diagnosis:
         A DSM-IV perspective* (pp. 289–307). Washington, D.C.: American
         Psychiatric Press.

Hunter, K.

1996 'Don't think zebras': Uncertainty, interpretation, and the place of paradox in clinical education. *Theoretical Medicine*, **17**, 225–241.

Ingleby, D.

1981 Understanding 'mental illness'. In D. Ingleby (Ed.). *Critical psychiatry* (pp. 23–71). Harmondsworth: Penguin.

1982 The social construction of mental illness. In P. W. G. Wright & A. Treacher (Eds.). *The problem of medical knowledge: Examining the social construction of medicine* (pp. 123–143). Edinburgh: University of Edinburgh Press.

Inkeles, A., & Smith, D. H.

1974 *Becoming modern: Individual change in six developing countries.* Cambridge, Massachusetts: Harvard University Press.

Jablensky, A., Sartorius, N., Cooper, J. E., Anker, M., Korten, A., & Bertelsen, A.

1994 Culture and schizophrenia. *British Journal of Psychiatry*, **165**, 434–436.

Jablensky, A., Sartorius, N., Ernberg, G., Anker, M., Korten, A., Cooper, J. E., Day, R., & Bertelsen, A.

1992 Schizophrenia: Manifestations, incidence and course in different cultures. A World Health Organization ten-country study. *Psychological Medicine, Monograph Supplement* **20**.

Jamison, K. R.

1995 *An unquiet mind.* New York: A. A. Knopf.

Janzen, J.

1978 *The quest for therapy in lower Zaire.* Berkeley: University of California Press.

Jenkins, J.

1988 Conceptions of schizophrenia as a problem of nerves: A cross-cultural comparison of Mexican-Americans and Anglo-Americans. *Social Science and Medicine*, **26**, 1233–1243.

Jenkins, J. H.

1991 Anthropology, expressed emotion, and schizophrenia. *Ethos*, **19**, 387–431.

Jenkins, J. H., & Karno, M.

1992 The meaning of expressed emotion: Theoretical issues raised by cross-cultural research. *American Journal of Psychiatry*, **149**, 9–21.

Jenkins, J. H., & Valiente, M.

1994 Bodily transactions of the passions: *el calor* among Salvadoran refugees. In T. J. Csordas (Ed.). *Embodiment and experience: The existential ground of culture and self* (pp. 163–182). Cambridge: Cambridge University Press.

Jewkes, R.

1984 The case for South Africa's expulsion from international psychiatry. New York: UN Center Against Apartheid.

Jones, J. S., Stein, D. S., Stanley, B., Guido, J. R., Winchel, R., & Stanley, M.
1994 Negative and depressive symptoms in suicidal schizophrenics.
Acta Psychiatrica Scandanavica, **89**, 81–87.

Jordan, G., & Weedon, C.
1995 *Cultural politics: Class, gender, race and the postmodern world*. Oxford:
Basil Blackwell.

Kareem, J., & Littlewood, R. (Eds.)
1992 *Intercultural therapy: Themes, interpretations and practice*. Oxford: Blackwell
Scientific Publications.

Karno, M., Jenkins, J. H., de la Selva, A., Santana, F., Telles, C., Lopez, S., & Mintz, J.
1987 Expressed emotion and schizophrenic outcome among Mexican-American
families. *The Journal of Nervous and Mental Disease*, **175**, 143–151.

Kaslow, N., Celano, M., & Dreelin, E. D.
1995 A cultural perspective on family theory and family therapy.
The Psychiatric Clinics of North America, **18**, 621–633.

Katon, W., & Kleinman, A.
1981 Clinical social science interventions in primary care: A review of doctor-
patient negotiation and other relevant social science concepts and
categories. In L. Eisenberg & A. Kleinman (Eds.). *The relevance of social
science for medicine* (pp. 253–278). Dordrecht: Reidel.

Katzenellenbogen, J. M., Matthews, C., & van der Walt, H.
1997 Community participation. In J. Katzenellenbogen, G. Joubert, & S. S.
Abdool-Karim (Eds.). *Epidemiology: A manual for Southern Africa* (pp. 34–46).
Cape Town: Oxford University Press.

Katzenellenbogen, J. M., Pick, W., Hoffman, M., & Weir, G.
1988 Community participation in the Mamre Community Health Project.
South African Medical Journal, **74**, 335–338.

Katzenellenbogen, J. M., Swartz L., & Hoffman, M. N.
1995 From research to service provision: The Mamre Community Health Project
– 7 years later. *South African Medical Journal*, **85**, 843–845.

Kennedy, J. G.
1987 *The flower of paradise*. Dordrecht: Reidel.

Kim, U., & Berry, J. W.
1993 Introduction. In U. Kim & J. W. Berry (Eds.). *Indigenous psychologies:
Research experience in cultural context* (pp. 1–29). Newbury Park: Sage.

Kirk, J.
1996 *Psychiatric, traditional and other interpretations of ukuthwetyulwa:
A witchcraft phenomenon in the Western Cape*. Unpublished M.A. thesis,
University of Cape Town.

Kirmayer, L. J.

1988   Mind and body as metaphors: Hidden values in biomedicine. In M. Lock & D. Gordon (Eds.). *Biomedicine examined* (pp. 57–93). Dordrecht: Kluwer.

1993   Healing and the invention of metaphor: The effectiveness of symbols revisited. *Culture, Medicine and Psychiatry*, **17**, 161–196.

Kirmayer, L. J., & Robbins, J. M.

1991   Three forms of somatization in primary care: Prevalence, co-occurrence, and socio-demographic characteristics. *Journal of Nervous and Mental Disease*, **179**, 647–655.

Kisely, S. R., & Goldberg, D. P.

1996   Physical and psychiatric comorbidity in general practice. *British Journal of Psychiatry*, **169**, 236–242.

Kleinman, A.

1977   Depression, somatization and the new cross-cultural psychiatry. *Social Science and Medicine*, **11**, 3–10.

1980   *Patients and healers in the context of culture*. Berkeley: University of California Press.

1986   *Social origins of distress and disease: Depression, neurasthenia, and pain in modern China*. New Haven and London: Yale University Press.

1988   *Rethinking psychiatry: From cultural category to personal experience*. New York: Free Press.

1995a   Do psychiatric disorders differ in different cultures? The methodological questions. In N. R. Goldberger & J. B. Veroff (Eds.). *The culture and psychology reader* (pp. 631–651). New York: New York University Press.

1995b   *Writing at the margin: Discourse between anthropology and medicine*. Berkeley: University of California Press.

Kleinman, A., Das, V., & Lock, M.

1996   Introduction (to the Winter 1996 issue: 'Social Suffering'). *Daedalus*, **125** (1), xi–xx.

Kleinman, A., Eisenberg, L., & Good, B. J.

1978   Culture, illness and care: Clinical lessons from anthropological and cross-cultural research. *Annals of Internal Medicine*, **88**, 251–258.

Kleinman, A., & Good, B. J.

1985b   Introduction: Culture and depression. In A. Kleinman & B. J. Good (Eds.). *Culture and depression: Studies in the anthropology and cross-cultural psychiatry of affect and disorder* (pp. 1–33). Berkeley: University of California Press.

Kleinman, A., & Good, B. J. (Eds.)

1985a   *Culture and depression: Studies in the anthropology and cross-cultural psychiatry of affect and disorder*. Berkeley: University of California Press.

Kleinman, A., & Kleinman, J.

1991 Suffering and its professional transformation: Towards an ethnography of interpersonal experience. *Culture, Medicine and Psychiatry*, **15**, 275–301.

1996 The appeal of experience; the dismay of images: Cultural appropriations of suffering in our times. *Daedalus*, **125** (1), xi–xx.

Koyama, T., & Yamashita, I.

1992 Biological markers of depression: WHO multi-center studies and future perspective. *Progress in Neuropsychopharmacology and Biological Psychiatry*, **16**, 791–796.

Kramer, P.

1993 *Listening to Prozac: A psychiatrist explores antidepressant drugs and the remaking of the self.* New York: Viking.

Kruger, D.

1974 Xhosa divining and psychotherapy — a reciprocal perspective. *Fort Hare Papers*, **6**, 37–46.

1978 Towards an understanding of the Xhosa diviner. *The Leech*, **48** (2), 7–13.

Kuipers, E.

1996 The management of difficult to treat patients with schizophrenia, using non-drug therapies. *British Journal of Psychiatry*, **169** (suppl. 31), 41–51.

Kuipers, L., & Bebbington, P.

1988 Expressed emotion research in schizophrenia: Theoretical and clinical implications. *Psychological Medicine*,**18**, 893–909.

Laing, R. D.

1960 *The divided self.* London: Tavistock.

Laing, R. D., & Esterson, A.

1964 *Sanity, madness and the family: Families of schizophrenics.* London: Tavistock.

Lambley, P.

1980 *The psychology of apartheid.* London: Secker & Warburg.

Lamla, C. M.

1976 *Present-day diviners (Ama-Gqira) in the Transkei.*Unpublished M.A. thesis, University of Fort Hare, Alice.

Lan, D.

1984 Spirit mediums and the authority to resist in the struggle for Zimbabwe. In *The societies of Southern Africa in the 19th and 20th centuries*, vol. 13. Collected seminar papers, **33**, 152–161. London: Institute of Commonwealth Studies, University of London.

Last, J. M.

1988 *Dictionary of epidemiology* (2nd edition). Oxford: Oxford University Press.

Last, M.
1992   The importance of knowing about not knowing: Observations from Hausaland. In S. Feierman & J. M. Janzen (Eds.). *The social basis of health and healing in Africa* (pp. 393 – 406). Berkeley: University of California Press.

Last, M., & Chavunduka, G. (Eds.)
1989   *The professionalisation of African medicine.* Manchester: Manchester University Press in association with the International African Institute.

Laubscher, B. J. F.
1937   *Sex, custom and psychopathology,* London: Routledge and Kegan Paul.

Lawrie, S. M., & Pelosi, A. J.
1995   Chronic fatigue syndrome in the community. Prevalence and associations. *British Journal of Psychiatry,* **166,** 793–797.

Lee, R. M.
1981   Structure and anti-structure in the culture-bound syndromes: The Malay case. *Culture, Medicine and Psychiatry,* **5,** 233–248.

Lee, S.
1996a   Cultures in psychiatric nosology: The CCMD-2-R and international classification of mental disorders. *Culture, Medicine and Psychiatry,* **20,** 421–472.
1996b   Reconsidering the status of anorexia nervosa as a culture-bound syndrome. *Social Science and Medicine,* **42,** 21–34.

Lee, S. G.
1969   Spirit possession among the Zulu. In J. Beattie & R. Middleton (Eds.). *Spirit mediumship and society in Africa* (pp. 128–156). London: Routledge and Kegan Paul.

Leff, J.
1981   *Psychiatry around the globe: A transcultural view.* New York: Marcel Dekker.
1988   *Psychiatry around the globe: A transcultural view* (2nd ed). London: Gaskell.

Leff, J., Sartorius, N., Jablensky, A., Korten, A., & Ernberg, G.
1992   The International Pilot Study of Schizophrenia: Five-year follow-up findings. *Psychological Medicine,* **22,** 131–145.

Leff, J., & Vaughn, C.
1985   *Expressed emotion in families: Its significance for mental illness.* New York: Guilford Press.

Leff, J., Wig, N. N., Bedi, H., Menon, D. K., Kuipers, L., Korten, A., Ernberg, G., Day, R., Sartorius, N., & Jablensky, A.
1990   Relatives' expressed emotion and the course of schizophrenia in Chandigarh: A two-year follow-up of a first-contact sample. *British Journal of Psychiatry,* **156,** 351–356.

Leff, J., Wig, N. N., Ghosh, A., Bedi, H., Menon, D. K., Kuipers, L., Korten, A., Ernberg, G., Day, R., Sartorius, N., & Jablensky, A.

1987   Expressed emotion and schizophrenia in North India. III. Influence of relatives' expressed emotion on the course of schizophrenia in Chandigarh. *British Journal of Psychiatry*, **151**, 166–173.

Levett, A.

1988   *Psychological trauma: Discourses on child sexual abuse.* Unpublished doctoral dissertation, University of Cape Town, Cape Town.

1995   Stigmatic factors in child sexual abuse and the violence of representation. *Psychology in Society*, **20**, 4–12.

Levett, A., Kottler, A., Walaza, N., Mabena, P., Leon, N., & Ngqakayi-Motaung, N.

1997   Pieces of mind: Traumatic effects of child sexual abuse among black South African women. In A. Levett, A. Kottler, E. Burman, & I. Parker (Eds.). *Culture, power and difference: Discourse analysis in South Africa* (pp. 125–138). London: Zed Books, and Cape Town: University of Cape Town Press.

LeVine, R., Dixon, S., LeVine, S., Richman, A., Liederman, P. H., Keefer, C. H., & Brazelton, T. B.

1994   *Child care and culture: Lessons from Africa.* Cambridge: Cambridge University Press.

Levy, J., Neutra, R., & Parker, D.

1987   *Hand trembling, frenzy witchcraft, and moth madness: A study of Navajo seizure disorders.* Tucson: University of Arizona Press.

Lewis-Fernández, R.

1996a   Cultural formulation of psychiatric diagnosis. *Culture, Medicine and Psychiatry*, **20**, 133–144.

1996b   Cultural formulation of psychiatric diagnosis. Case No. 02: Diagnosis and treatment of nervios and ataques in a female Puerto Rican migrant. *Culture, Medicine and Psychiatry*, **20**, 155–163.

Lewis-Fernández, R., & Kleinman, A.

1995   Cultural psychiatry: theoretical, clinical, and research issues. *The Psychiatric Clinics of North America*, **18**, 433–448.

Lex, B. W.

1995   Alcohol and other psychoactive substance dependence in women and men. In M. V. Seeman (Ed). *Gender and psychopathology* (pp. 311–358). Washington, D.C.: American Psychiatric Press.

Lifton, R. J.

1967   *Death in life: Survivors of Hiroshima.* New York: Random House.

1986   *The Nazi doctors: Medical killing and the psychology of genocide.* New York: Basic Books.

Light, D.
1980   *Becoming psychiatrists: The professional transformation of the self.*
        New York: Norton.

Lim, R. F., & Lin, K.-M.
1996   Cultural formulation of psychiatric diagnosis. Case No. 03: Psychosis
        following *Qi-gong* in a Chinese immigrant. *Culture, Medicine and
        Psychiatry,* **20,** 369–378.

Lipsedge, M., & Littlewood, R.
1997   Psychopathology and its public sources: From a provisional typology to a
        dramaturgy of domestic sieges. *Anthropology and Medicine,* **4,** 25–43.

Littlewood, R.
1988   Community initiated research: A study in psychiatrists' conceptualisations
        of 'cannabis psychosis'. *Bulletin of the Royal College of Psychiatrists,*
        12, 486–488.

1990   From categories to contexts: A decade of the 'new cross-cultural
        psychiatry'. *British Journal of Psychiatry,* **156,** 308–327.

1992a   How universal is something we can call therapy? In J. Kareem & R.
        Littlewood (Eds.). *Intercultural therapy: Themes, interpretations and practice*
        (pp. 38–56). Oxford: Blackwell Scientific Publications.

1992b   Towards an intercultural therapy. In J. Kareem & R. Littlewood (Eds.).
        Intercultural therapy: Themes, interpretations and practice (pp. 3–13).
        Oxford: Blackwell Scientific Publications.

1994   Symptoms, struggles and functions: What does the overdose represent?
        In M. McDonald (Ed.). *Gender, drink and drugs* (pp. 77–98). Oxford: Berg
        Publishers.

1996   Comments on culture-bound syndromes: I. In J. E. Mezzich, A. Kleinman,
        H. Fabrega, Jr., & D. L. Parron (Eds.). *Culture and diagnosis: A DSM-IV
        perspective* (pp. 309–312). Washington, D.C.: American Psychiatric Press.

Littlewood, R., & Lipsedge, M.
1986   The 'culture-bound syndromes' of the dominant culture: Culture,
        psychopathology and biomedicine. In J. L. Cox (Ed.). *Transcultural
        psychiatry* (pp. 253–273). London: Croom Helm.

1987   The butterfly and the serpent: Culture, psychopathology and biomedicine.
        Culture, Medicine and Psychiatry, **11,** 289–335.

1988   Psychiatric illness among British Afro-Caribbeans. *British Medical Journal,*
        296, 950–951.

1989   *Aliens and alienists: Ethnic minorities and psychiatry* (2nd ed.). London:
        Unwin Hyman.

1997   *Aliens and alienists: Ethnic minorities and psychiatry* (3rd ed.). London:
        Routledge.

Lock, M.
1987   DSM-III as a culture-bound construct: Commentary on culture-bound
        syndromes and international disease classifications. *Culture, Medicine and
        Psychiatry*, **11**, 35–42.
1989   Words of fear, words of power: Nerves and the awakening of political
        consciousness. *Medical Anthropology*, **11**, 79–90.
1990   On being ethnic: The politics of identity breaking and making in Canada,
        or *nevra* on Sunday. *Culture, Medicine and Psychiatry*, **14**, 237–254.

Lock, M., & Gordon, D. (Eds.)
1988   *Biomedicine examined*. Dordrecht: Kluwer.

Lock, M., & Lella, J.
1986   Reforming medical education: Towards a broadening of attitudes.
        In S. McHugh & T.M. Vallis (Eds.). *Illness behaviour: A multidisciplinary model*
        (pp. 47–58). New York: Plenum Press.

Lock, M., & Scheper-Hughes, N.
1990   A critical-interpretive approach in medical anthropology: Rituals and
        routines of discipline and dissent. In T. M. Johnson & C. E. Sargent (Eds.).
        Medical anthropology: Contemporary theory and method (pp. 47–72).
        New York: Praeger.

Louw, J.
1986   *This is thy work: A contextual history of applied psychology and labour in South
        Africa*. Unpublished doctoral dissertation, University of Leiden.

Louw, J., Katzenellenbogen, J., & Carolissen, R.
1995   Community health needs, community participation and evaluation.
        Evaluation and Programme Planning, **74**, 335–338.

Low, S. M.
1985   Culturally interpreted symptoms or culture-bound syndromes:
        A cross-cultural review of nerves. *Social Science and Medicine*, **21**, 187–196.
1988   Medical practice in response to a folk illness: The treatment of
        nervios in Costa Rica. In M. Lock & D. Gordon (Eds.). *Biomedicine examined*
        (pp. 415–438). Dordrecht: Kluwer.
1994   Embodied metaphors: Nerves as lived experience. In T. J. Csordas (Ed.).
        Embodiment and experience: The existential ground of culture and self
        (pp. 139–162). Cambridge: Cambridge University Press.

Lucas, R. H., & Barrett, R.
1995   Interpreting culture and psychopathology: Primitivist themes in
        cross-cultural debate. *Culture, Medicine and Psychiatry*, **19**, 287–326.

Luiz, H. A.
1981   Profile of a psychiatric clinic in Soweto. *Transactions of the College of
        Medicine of South Africa*, **25**, Supplementum, 187–190.

Lund, C.

1994   *Xhosa speaking schizophrenic patients' experience of their condition: Psychosis
        or amafufunyana?* Unpublished psychology honours research project,
        University of Cape Town.

Lutz, C.

1985   Depression and the translation of emotional worlds. In A. Kleinman &
        B. Good (Eds.). *Culture and depression: Studies in the anthropology and
        cross-cultural psychiatry of affect and disorder* (pp. 63–100). Berkeley:
        University of California Press.

Lynn, S. J., & Rhue, J. W.

1994   Introduction: Dissociation and dissociative disorders in perspective.
        In S. J. Lynn & J. W. Rhue (Eds.). *Dissociation: Clinical and theoretical
        perspectives* (pp. 1–11). New York: Guilford Press.

Lyon, M. L.

1996   C. Wright Mills meets Prozac: The relevance of 'social emotion' to the
        sociology of health and illness. In V. James & J. Gabe (Eds.). *Health and the
        sociology of emotions* (pp. 55–78). Oxford: Blackwell Publishers.

Mama, A.

1995   *Beyond the masks: Race, gender and subjectivity.* London: Routledge.

Manganyi, N. C.

1973   *Being black in the world.* Johannesburg: Sprocas/Ravan.

1991   *Treachery and innocence: Psychology and racial difference in South Africa.*
        Johannesburg: Ravan.

Marcos, L.

1979   Effects of interpreters on the evaluation of psychopathology in
        non-English speaking patients. *American Journal of Psychiatry, 136,* 171–175.

Marks, S.

1994   *Divided sisterhood: Race, class and gender in the South African nursing profession.*
        New York: St Martin's Press.

Martin, G., Steyn, K., & Yach, D.

1992   Beliefs about smoking and health and attitudes towards tobacco control
        measures. *South African Medical Journal, 82,* 241–245.

Mattes, J. A., & Amsell, L.

1993   The dexamethasone suppression test as an indication of depression in
        patients with mental retardation. *American Journal of Mental Retardation,
        98,* 354–359.

Matthews, C., Van der Walt, H., & Barron, P.

1994   A shotgun marriage: Qualitative evaluation of a community health worker
        project in Khayelitsha. *South African Medical Journal, 84,* 659–663.

Maw, A.
1996   *The consultation relationship as a complex partnership.* Unpublished M.A. thesis, University of Cape Town.

Mazel, J.
1981   *Beverly Hills diet.* New York: Macmillan.

McCallum, T. G.
1994   *White woman witch doctor: Tales from the African life of Rae Graham.* Sandton, South Africa: Struik Book Distributors.

McCulloch, J.
1995   *Colonial psychiatry and 'the African mind'.* Cambridge: Cambridge University Press.

McDonald, M.
1994   Introduction: A social-anthroplogical view of gender, drink and drugs. In M. McDonald (Ed.). *Gender, drink and drugs* (pp. 1–31). Oxford: Berg Publishers.

McGoldrick, M., Pearce, J. K., & Giordano, J. (Eds.)
1982   *Ethnicity and family therapy.* New York: Guilford Press.

McGovern D., & Cope, R.
1987   The complusory detention of males of different ethnic groups. *British Journal of Psychiatry,* **150,** 505–512.

McQueen, A. H., & Swartz, L.
1995   Reports of the experience of epilepsy in a rural South African village. *Social Science and Medicine,* **21,** 859–865.

McQueen, A. H., Swartz, L., & Pefile, L. L.
1995   Epilepsy and psychosocial adjustment: A selective review. *South African Journal of Psychology,* **24,** 207–210.

Mdleleni, T.
1986   *Amafufunyane spirit possession and faith healing practices: A pilot study.* Unpublished psychology honours research project, University of Cape Town.

Mdleleni, T. N.
1990   *Cultural construction of psychiatric illness: A case of amafufunyane.* Unpublished M.A. thesis, University of Cape Town.

Menuck, M., Legault, S., Schmidt, P., & Remington, G.
1989   The nosologic status of the remitting atypical psychoses. *Comprehensive Psychiatry,* **30,** 53–73.

Merskey, H., & Shafran, B.
1986   Political hazards in the diagnosis of 'sluggish schizophrenia'. *British Journal of Psychiatry,* **148,** 247–256.

Mezzich, J. E., Kleinman, A., Fabrega, H., Jr., & Parron, D. L. (Eds.)
1996   *Culture and diagnosis: A DSM-IV perspective.* Washington, D.C.: American Psychiatric Press.

Miller, T., & Swartz, L.
1990a   Access to psychiatric resources: The case of Mamre. Presented at the Association for Sociology in Southern Africa Conference, Stellenbosch, July.
1990b   Clinical psychology in general hospital settings: Issues in interprofessional relationships. *Professional Psychology: Research and Practice,* **21**, 48–53.
1991   Integration or marginalization: Clinical psychology as a strategy for dealing with psychosocial issues in a South African neurosurgery ward. *Sociology of Health and Illness,* **13**, 293–309.
1992   Psychology and epidemiology: An uncomfortable alliance? *South African Journal of Psychology,* **22**, 52–58.

Miller, T., Swartz, L., & Rumble, S.
1991   Psychological factors in primary health care in Mamre. Presented at the Epidemiological Society of South Africa Conference, University of the Western Cape, July 1991.

Mills, J.
1983   *Health, healing and dis-ease in a South African township.* Unpublished master's thesis, University of Cape Town.
1985   The possession state *intwaso*: An anthropological re-appraisal. *South African Journal of Sociology,* **16**, 9–13.

Milner, G., & Hayes, G.
1988   Psychiatric illness among British Afro-Caribbeans (letter). *British Medical Journal,* **296**, 1333.

Minde, M.
1974a   History of mental health services in South Africa. Part I. In the days of the Dutch East India Company. *South African Medical Journal,* **48**, 1270–1271.
1974b   History of mental health services in South Africa. Part II. During the British occupation. *South African Medical Journal,* **48**, 1629–1632.
1974c   History of mental health services in South Africa. Part III. The Cape Province. *South African Medical Journal,* **48**, 2230–2234.
1974d   History of mental health services in South Africa. Part IV. The Orange Free State. *South African Medical Journal,* **48**, 2327–2330.
1975a   History of mental health services in South Africa. Part V. Natal. *South African Medical Journal,* **49**, 322–326.
1975b   History of mental health services in South Africa. Part VI. The Transvaal. *South African Medical Journal,* **49**, 367–374.
1975c   History of mental health services in South Africa. Part VII. Services since Union. *South African Medical Journal,* **49**, 405–409.

1975d   History of mental health services in South Africa. Part VIII. Services for
          epileptics. *South African Medical Journal*, **49**, 1568–1572.
1975e   History of mental health services in South Africa. Part IX. The protection
          and care of the feebleminded. *South African Medical Journal*, **49**, 1716–1720.
1975f   History of mental health services in South Africa. Part X. Institutions for
          defectives. *South African Medical Journal*, **49**, 1890–1894.
1975g   History of mental health services in South Africa. Part XI. Services for
          alcoholics. *South African Medical Journal*, **49**, 2197–2202.
1975h   History of mental health services in South Africa. Part XII. Services for
          criminals, delinquents and psychopaths. *South African Medical Journal*,
          49, 2265–2270.
1976   History of mental health services in South Africa. Part XIII. The National
          Council for Mental Health. *South African Medical Journal*, **50**, 1452–1456.
1977a   History of mental health services in South Africa. Part XIV. Psychiatric
          education. *South African Medical Journal*, **51**, 210–214.
1977b   History of mental health services in South Africa. Part XV. The future of
          mental health services. *South African Medical Journal*, **51**, 549–553.

Mizrahi, T.
1987   Getting rid of patients: Contradictions in the socialization of internists to
          the doctor-patient relationship. *Sociology of Health and Illness*, 7, 214–235.

Mkhwanazi, I. M.
1986   *An investigation of the therapeutic methods of Zulu diviners.* Unpublished M.A.
          thesis, University of South Africa, Pretoria.

Montagne, M.
1991   The culture of long-term tranquilliser users. In J. Gabe (Ed.).
          Understanding tranquilliser use: The role of the social sciences (pp. 48–68).
          London: Tavistock/ Routledge.

Mossman, D.
1997   Deinstitutionalization, homelessness and the myth of psychiatric
          abandonment: A structural anthropology perspective. *Social Science and
          Medicine*, **44**, 71–83.

Mudford, O. C., Barrera, F. J., Murray, A., Boundy, K., Caldwell, K., & Goldberg, B.
1995   The dexamethasone suppression test and the diagnosis of depression in
          adults with severe and profound developmental disabilities. *Journal of
          Intellectual Disability Research*, **39**, 275–283.

Muller, L.
1994   *'Poor' clinical interpreting for 'good' psychiatric practice: Xhosa interpreting
          within a diagnostic interview in an acute admissions unit.* Unpublished
          psychology honours research project, University of Cape Town.

Murphy, H. B. M.
1977   Transcultural psychiatry should begin at home. *Psychological Medicine*,
           7, 369–371.

Murphy, H. B. M., & Raman, A. C.
1971   The chronicity of schizophrenia in indigenous tropical peoples: Results of
           a twelve-year follow-up survey in Mauritius. *British Journal of Psychiatry*,
           118, 489–497.

Murphy, J. M.
1976   Psychiatric labelling in cross-cultural perspective. *Science*, 191, 1019–1028.

Mustafa, G.
1991   Problems in psychiatry services in Sub-Sahara African countries.
           In S. O. Okpaku (Ed.). *Mental health in Africa and the Americas today*
           (pp. 387-393). Nashville: Crisolith Books.

Myers, J. E., White, N., & Cornell, J. E.
1982   Prevalence of hypertension in semi-skilled manual workers. *South African
           Medical Journal*, 62, 894–898.

Nations, M. K., Camino, L. A., & Walker, F. B.
1985   Hidden popular illnesses in primary care: Residents' recognition and
           clinical implications. *Culture, Medicine and Psychiatry*, 9, 223–240.
1988   'Nerves': Folk idiom for anxiety and depression? *Social Science and
           Medicine*, 26, 1245–1259.

Ngubane, H.
1977   *Body and mind in Zulu medicine: An ethnography of health and disease
           in Nyuswa-Zulu thought and practice.* London: Academic Press.

Nicholas, L. J. (Ed.)
1993   *Psychology and oppression: Critiques and proposals.* Johannesburg: Skotaville.

Nicholas, L. J., & Cooper, S. (Eds.)
1990   *Psychology and apartheid: Essays on the struggle for psychology and the mind in
           South Africa.* Johannesburg: Vision / Madiba.

Nichter, M., & Cartwright, E.
1991   Saving the children for the tobacco industry. *Medical Anthropology
           Quarterly*, 5, 236–256.

Obeyesekere, G.
1985   Depression, Buddhism and the work of culture in Sri Lanka. In A.
           Kleinman & B. Good (Eds.). *Culture and depression: Studies in the anthropology
           and cross-cultural psychiatry of affect and disorder* (pp. 134–152). Berkeley:
           University of California Press.

O'Connell, M. C.
1980   The aetiology of thwasa. *Psychotherapeia*, 6 (4), 18–23.

1982   Spirit possession and role stress among the Xesibe of Eastern Transkei. *Ethnology*, **21**, 21–37.

Odejide, A. O., Oyewunmi, L. K., & Ohaeri, J. U.
1989   Psychiatry in Africa: An overview. *American Journal of Psychiatry*, **146**, 708–716.

Olwig, K. F., & Hastrup, K. (Eds.)
1997   *Siting culture: The shifting anthropological object*. London: Routledge.

Oppenheimer, E.
1991   Drug misuse in the community: Meeting the need. In D. H. Bennett & H. L. Freeman (Eds.). *Community psychiatry: The principles* (pp. 337–360). Edinburgh: Churchill Livingstone.

Orford, J.
1985   *Excessive appetites: A psychological view of addictions*. Chichester: John Wiley and Sons.
1991   Alcohol problems in the community. In D. H. Bennett & H. L. Freeman (Eds.). *Community psychiatry: The principles* (pp. 297–336). Edinburgh: Churchill Livingstone.

Orley, J.
1970   *Culture and mental illness*. Nairobi: East African Publishing House.

Orley, J., & Isaac, M.
1997   Review of R. Desjarlais, L. Eisenberg, B. Good, & A. Kleinman (1995). *World mental health: Problems and priorities in low-income countries*. New York and Oxford: Oxford University Press. *Transcultural Psychiatry*, **34**, 141–145.

Orley, J., & Wing, J. K.
1979   Psychiatric disorder in two African villages. *Archives of General Psychiatry*, **36**, 513–526.

Owens, I.
1996   *Reconstruction of the nation: Embracing the multiple paths of healing*. Unpublished psychology honours research project, University of Cape Town.

Parker, G., Hadzi-Pavolvic, D., Hickie, I., Brodaty, H., Boyce, P., Mitchell, P., & Wilhelm, K.
1995   Sub-typing depression, III. Development of a clinical algorithm for melancholia and comparison with other diagnostic measures. *Psychological Medicine*, **25**, 833–840.

Parry, C. D. H.
1996   A review of psychiatric epidemiology in Africa: Strategies for improving validity when using instruments transculturally. *Transcultural Psychiatric Research Review*, **33**, 173–178.

1997   Alcohol, drug abuse and public health in South Africa: Policy considerations.
            In D. Foster, M. Freeman, & Y. Pillay (Eds.). *Mental health policy issues for
            South Africa* (pp. 290–315). Cape Town: MASA Multimedia.

Parry, C. D. H., & Bennetts, A. L.
in press   Alcohol policy and public health in South Africa. Cape Town: Oxford
            University Press.

Parry, C. D. H., & Swartz, L.
1997   Psychiatric epidemiology. In J. Katzenellenbogen, G. Joubert, & S. S.
            Abdool-Karim (Eds.). *Epidemiology: A manual for Southern Africa*
            (pp. 230–242). Cape Town: Oxford University Press.

Patel, V., & Winston, M.
1994   'Universality of mental illness' revisited: Assumptions, artefacts and new
            directions. *British Journal of Psychiatry*, **165**, 437–440.

Pedersen, P. (Ed.)
in press   *Multiculturalism as a fourth force*. New York: Taylor & Francis.

Peltzer, K.
1995   *Psychology and health in African cultures: Examples of ethnopsychotherapeutic
            practice*. Frankfurt: IKO — Verlag für Interkulturelle Kommunikation.

Peltzer, K., & Ebigbo, P. (Eds.)
1989   *Clinical psychology in Africa*. Enugu: Working Group of Psychology in Africa.

Pena, J. M., & Koss-Chioino, J. D.
1992   Cultural sensitivity in drug treatment research with African American
            males. In J. E. Trimble, C. S. Bolek, & S. J. Niemcryk (Eds.). *Ethnic and
            multicultural drug use: Perspectives on current research* (pp. 157–179).
            Binghamton, New York: Harrington Park Press.

Penn, D. L., & Mueser, K. T.
1996   Research update on the psychosocial treatment of schizophrenia.
            American Journal of Psychiatry, **153**, 607–617.

Petersen, I., Bhagwanjee, A., Parekh, A., Parukh, Z., & Subedar, H. (Eds.)
1996   *Developing primary mental health care systems in South Africa: The case of
            KwaDedangendlale*. Durban: The Community Mental Health Project,
            Department of Psychology, University of Durban-Westville.

Petersen, I., & Parekh, A.
1996   Understanding minor psychiatric disorders. In I. Petersen, A. Bhagwanjee,
            A. Parekh, Z. Parukh., & H. Subedar (Eds.). *Developing primary mental
            health care systems in South Africa: The case of KwaDedangendlale* (pp. 67–73).
            Durban: The Community Mental Health Project, Department of
            Psychology, University of Durban-Westville.

Ponterotto, J. G., Casas, J. M., Suzuki, L. A., & Alexander, C. M. (Eds.)
1995   *Handbook of multicultural counseling*. Thousand Oaks, California: Sage.

Potgieter, W.
1986   Die werksku kleurlingman: 'n Psigodiagnostiese ondersoek. Unpublished
        master's thesis, Potchefstroomse Universiteit vir Christelike Hoër
        Onderwys, Potchefstroom.

Prather, J. E.
1991   Decoding advertising: The role of communication studies in explaining the
        popularity of minor tranquillisers. In J. Gabe (Ed.). *Understanding
        tranquilliser use: The role of the social sciences* (pp. 112–135). London:
        Tavistock/ Routledge.

Prince, R.
1985   The concept of culture-bound syndromes: Anorexia nervosa and brain-fag.
        Social Science and Medicine, **21**, 197–203.

Prince, R., & Tcheng-Laroche, F.
1987   Culture-bound syndromes and international disease classifications.
        Culture, Medicine and Psychiatry, **11**, 3–20.

Putnam, F. W.
1993   Dissociative phenomena. In D. Spiegel (Ed.). *Dissociative disorders:
        A clinical review* (pp. 1–16). Lutherville, USA: Sidran Press.

Ramphele, M.
1993   *A bed called home: Life in the migrant labour hostels of Cape Town*. Cape Town:
        David Philip.
1996   Political widowhood in South Africa: The embodiment of ambiguity.
        Daedalus, **125** (1), 99–117.

Ray, L.
1991   The political economy of long-term minor tranquilliser use. In J. Gabe
        (Ed.). *Understanding tranquilliser use: The role of the social sciences*
        (pp. 136–161). London: Tavistock/ Routledge.

Reeler, A. P.
1987   Psychological disorders in Africa II: Clinical issues. *Central African Journal
        of Medicine*, **33**, 15–19.

Reynolds, J.
1990   *Nerves in Mamré: Somatisation as communication*. Unpublished psychology
        honours research project, University of Cape Town.

Reynolds, J., & Swartz, L.
1993   Professional constructions of a 'lay' illness: 'Nerves' in a rural 'coloured'
        community in South Africa. *Social Science and Medicine*, **36**, 657–663.

Reynolds, P.
1996   *Traditional healers and childhood in Zimbabwe.* Athens, Ohio: University of
          Ohio Press.

Rhodes, L. A.
1991   *Emptying beds: The work of a psychiatric emergency psychiatric unit.*
          Berkeley: University of California Press.

Ribeiro, S. C., Tandon, R., Grunhaus, L., & Greden, J. F.
1993   The DST as a predictor of outcome in depression: A meta-analysis.
          American Journal of Psychiatry, **150,** 1618–1629.

Ritenbaugh, C.
1982   Obesity as a culture-bound syndrome. *Culture, Medicine and Psychiatry,*
          6, 347–361.

Ritenbaugh, C., Shisslak, C., Teufel, N., & Leonard-Green, T. K.
1996   A cross-cultural review of eating disorders in regard to DSM-IV.
          In J. E. Mezzich, A. Kleinman, H. Fabrega, Jr., & D. L. Parron (Eds.).
          Culture and diagnosis: A DSM-IV perspective (pp. 171–185). Washington, D.C.:
          American Psychiatric Press.

Robertson, B.
1996   *Handbook of child psychiatry for primary care.* Cape Town: Oxford University
          Press.

Robins, L. N., & Reiger, D. A. (Eds.)
1992   *Psychiatric disorders in America: The Epidemiologic Catchment Area Study.*
          New York: The Free Press.

Rocha-Silva, L.
1991   *Alcohol and other drug use by Blacks resident in selected areas in the RSA.*
          Pretoria: Human Sciences Research Council.
1997   Drug use in South Africa. Paper presented at a workshop organized by the
          South African Institute of International Affairs (SAIIA) on The Illegal Drug
          Trade in Southern Africa, Jan Smuts House, University of South Africa,
          5–6 June.

Rocha-Silva, L., De Miranda, S., & Tshabalala, P.
1995   Silent threat: Drug use amongst South Africa's black youth. *HSRC Update,*
          5(4), 8–13.

Rogers, C.
1961   *On becoming a person.* Boston: Houghton Mifflin.

Rogers, P.
1992   *Explanatory models of illness amongst primary health care users in Mamre.*
          Unpublished M.A. thesis, University of Cape Town.

Roth, L., & Swartz, L.
1992   The integration of two psychotherapeutic units: Staff experiences of the
        first six months. *South African Journal of Occupational Therapy*, **22** (2), 6–11.

Rottanburg, D.
1982   *A toxicological study of acute psychoses in Cape Coloured males with special
        reference to the cannabinoids.* Unpublished M.A. thesis, University of
        Cape Town.

Rottanburg, D., Robins, A.H., Ben-Arie, O., Teggin, A.F., & Elk, R.
1982   Cannabis-associated psychosis with hypomanic features. *The Lancet*,
        2, 1364–1366.

Rousseau, C.
1995   The mental health of refugee children. *Transcultural Psychiatric Research
        Review*, **32**, 299–331.

Rubel, A. J., O'Nell, C. W., & Collado-Ardón, R.
1984   *Susto: A folk illness.* Berkeley: University of California Press.

Rumble, S., Swartz, L., Parry, C., & Zwarenstein, M.
1996   Prevalence of psychiatric morbidity in the adult population of a rural
        South African village. *Psychological Medicine*, **26**, 997–1007.

Sartorius, N.
1992   Comment on 'Prognosis for schizophrenia in the Third World', by Alex
        Cohen. *Culture, Medicine and Psychiatry*, **16**, 81–84.

Sartorius, N., Jablensky, A., Korten, A., Ernberg, G., Naker, M., Cooper, J. E.,
& Day, R.
1986   Early manifestations and first-contact incidence of schizophrenia in
        different cultures: A preliminary report on the initial evaluation phase of
        the WHO collaborative study on Determinants of Outcome of Severe
        Mental Disorders. *Psychological Medicine*, **16**, 909–928.

Sashidharan, S. P.
1981   South Africa and the Royal College of Psychiatrists. *The Lancet*, **2**, 1049.

Sashidharan, S. P., Cox, J.L., Orley, J., Shoenberg, E., Webster, J., Rack, P., Littlewood,
R., Lipsedge, M.S., & Davis, B.
1982   South Africa and the Royal College of Psychiatrists. *The Lancet*, **2**, 497–498.

Sashidharan, S. P., & Francis, E.
1993   Epidemiology, ethnicity and schizophrenia. In W. I. U. Ahmad (Ed.).
        'Race' and health in contemporary Britain (pp. 96–113). Buckingham:
        Open University Press.

Sashidharan, S. P., & Lipsedge, M.
1986   Schizophrenia and ethnicity (letter). *British Journal of Psychiatry*, **148**, 484.

Sashidharan, S. P., & Platt, S.
1987   Comment on 'The state of psychiatry in South Africa today' by John
        Dommisse. *Social Science and Medicine*, **24**, 758–760.

Scheper-Hughes, N.
1992   *Death without weeping: The violence of everyday life in Brazil.* Berkeley:
        University of California Press.

Scheper-Hughes, N., & Lock, M.
1987   The mindful body: A prolegomenon to future work in medical anthropology.
        Medical Anthropology Quarterly, **2**, 6–41.

Schoeman, J. B.
1989   Psigopatologie by tradisionele swart Suid-Afrikaners. In D. A. Louw (Ed.).
        Suid-Afrikaanse handboek van abnormale gedrag (pp. 448–470).
        Johannesburg: Southern.

Schweitzer, R.D.
1977   *Categories of experience amongst the Xhosa: A psychological study.* Unpublished
        M.A. thesis, Rhodes University, Grahamstown.

Scott, J.
1985   *Weapons of the weak: Everyday forms of peasant resistance.* New Haven and
        London: Yale University Press.

Seeman, M. V. (Ed.)
1995   *Gender and psychopathology.* Washington, D.C.: American Psychiatric Press.

Shanks, M. F., & Ho-Yen, D. O.
1995   A clinical study of chronic fatigue syndrome. *British Journal of Psychiatry*,
        166, 798–801.

Sharp, J.
1980   Can we study ethnicity? A critique of fields of study in South African
        anthropology. *Social Dynamics*, **6**, 1–16.
1988   Introduction: Constructing social reality. In E. Boonzaier & J. Sharp (Eds.).
        South African keywords: Uses and abuses of political concepts (pp 1–16).
        Cape Town: David Philip.

Sharpe, M., Hawton, K., Simkin, S., Surawy, C., Hackmann, A., Klimes, I., Peto, T.,
Warrell, D., & Seagroatt, V.
1996   Cognitive behaviour therapy for the chronic fatigue syndrome:
        A randomised controlled trial. *British Medical Journal*, **312** (7022), 22–26.

Shaw, J., Kennedy, S. H., & Joffe, R. T.
1995   Gender differences in mood disorders: A clinical focus. In M. V. Seeman
        (Ed.). *Gender and psychopathology* (pp. 89–111). Washington, D.C.:
        American Psychiatric Press.

Shweder, R. A.

1977   Likeness and likelihood in everyday thought: Magical thinking in
judgements about personality. *Current Anthropology*, **18**, 637–658.

1984   Anthropology's romantic rebellion against the Enlightenment, or There's
more to thinking than reason and evidence. In R. A. Shweder & R. A.
LeVine (Eds.). *Culture theory: Essays on mind, self and emotion* (pp. 27–66).
Cambridge: Cambridge University Press.

1990   Cultural psychology — what is it? In J. W. Stigler, R. A. Shweder, & G. Herdt
(Eds.). *Cultural psychology: Essays on comparative human development*
(pp. 1–43). New York: Cambridge University Press.

Shweder, R. A., & Bourne, E.

1982,   Does the concept of the person vary cross-culturally? In A. Marsella &
G. M. White (Eds.). *Cultural conceptions of mental health and therapy*
(pp. 97–137). Dordrecht: Reidel.

Sifneos, P. E.

1973   The prevalence of 'alexithymic' characteristics in psychosomatic patients.
Psychotherapy and Psychosomatics, **22**, 255–262.

Sijuwola, O. A.

1995   Culture, religion and mental illness in Nigeria. In I. Al-Issa (Ed.).
Handbook of culture and mental illness: An international perspective (pp. 65–72).
Madison: International Universities Press.

Silove, D., Sinnerbrink, I., Field, A., Manicavasagar, V., & Steel, Z.

1997   Anxiety, depression and PTSD in asylum-seekers: Associations with
pre-migration trauma and post-migration stressors. *British Journal of
Psychiatry*, **170**, 351–357.

Simons, R. C., & Hughes, C.C. (Eds.)

1985   *The culture-bound syndromes: Folk illnesses of psychiatric and anthropological
interest*. Dordrecht: Reidel.

Sinason, V.

1992   *Mental handicap and the human condition: New approaches from the Tavistock*.
London: Free Association Books.

Sinason, V. (Ed.)

1994   *Treating survivors of satanist abuse*. London: Routledge.

in press *Memory in dispute*. London: Karnac Books.

Sinzingre, N., & Zempléni, A.

1992   Causality of disease among the Senufo. In S. Feierman, & J. M. Janzen (Eds.).
The social basis of health and healing in Africa (pp. 315–338). Berkeley:
University of California Press.

Skinner, D., & Swartz, L.

1989   The effect of a parent's detention on the preschool child: A preliminary South African study of caregivers' reports. *Journal of Child Psychology and Psychiatry*, **30**, 243–259.

Slovo, G.

1997   *Every secret thing: My family, my country.* London: Little, Brown and Company.

Soni, S., Keane, V., & Soni, S. D.

1992   Dexamethasone suppression test and response to antidepressants in depressed mentally handicapped subjects. *Journal of Intellectual Disability Research*, **36**, 425–433.

Spanos, N. P., & Burgess, C.

1994   Hypnosis and multiple personality disorder: A sociocognitive perpective. In S. J. Lynn & J. W. Rhue (Eds.). *Dissociation: Clinical and theoretical perspectives* (pp. 136–155). New York: Guilford Press.

Spiegel, A. D., & Mehlwana, A. M.

1997   *Family as social network: Kinship and sporadic migrancy in the Western Cape's Khayelitsha.* Report no. HG/MF – 31. Pretoria: HSRC.

Spiegel, D.

1993a   Dissociation and trauma. In D. Spiegel (Ed.). *Dissociative disorders: A clinical review* (pp. 117–131). Lutherville, USA: Sidran Press.

1993b   Dissociative disorders: Preface. In D. Spiegel (Ed.). *Dissociative disorders: A clinical review* (pp. ix–x). Lutherville, USA: Sidran Press.

Spiro, M.

1991   *Illness models of relatives of African psychiatric patients: Implications for a family-based service.* Unpublished M.A. thesis, University of Cape Town.

Spivak, G. C.

1990   *The post-colonial critic: Interviews, strategies, dialogue* (Ed. S. Harasym). New York: Routledge.

Steinberg, D.

1992   Interprofessional consultation: Creative approaches in therapeutic work across cultures. In J. Kareem & R. Littlewood (Eds.). *Intercultural therapy: Themes, interpretations and practice* (pp. 59–73). Oxford: Blackwell Scientific Publications.

Sterling, C., & Lazarus, R.

1995   *Teaching lay-counsellors: A manual for trainers.* Cape Town: University of Cape Town Child Guidance Clinic.

Stone, A., Pinder-Hughes, C., Spurlock, J., & Weinberg, D.

1979   *See* Committee to Visit South Africa.

Straker, G.

1988   Posttraumatic stress disorder: A reaction to state-sponsored child abuse. *Child Abuse and Neglect*, **12**, 383–395.

1992   *Faces in the revolution: The psychological effects of violence on township youth in South Africa.* Cape Town: David Philip.

Straker, G., & the Sanctuaries Counselling Team

1987   The continuous traumatic stress syndrome: The single therapeutic interview. *Psychology in Society*, **8**, 48–78.

Sugarman, P. A., & Craufurd, D.

1994   Schizophrenia in the Afro-Caribbean community. *British Journal of Psychiatry*, **164**, 474–480.

Sullivan, M.

1986   In what sense is contemporary medicine dualistic? *Culture, Medicine and Psychiatry*, **10**, 331–350.

Sumba, R. O.

1991   Cannabis psychosis: Facts and myth. In S. O. Okpaku (Ed.). *Mental health in Africa and the Americas today* (pp. 339–346). Nashville: Crisolith Books.

Surawy, C., Hackmann, A., Hawton, K., & Sharpe, M.

1995   Chronic fatigue syndrome: A cognitive approach. *Behaviour Research and Therapy*, **33**, 535–544.

Susser, E., Finnerty, M. T., & Sohler, N.

1996   Acute psychoses: A proposed diagnosis for ICD-11 and DSM-V. *Psychiatric Quarterly*, **67** (3), 165–176.

Susser, E., Varma, V. K., Malhotra, S., Conover, S., & Amador, X. F.

1995   Delineation of acute and transient psychotic disorders in a developing country setting. *British Journal of Psychiatry*, **167**, 216–219.

Susser, E., & Wanderling, J.

1994   Epidemiology of nonaffective acute remitting psychosis: Sex and sociocultural setting. *Archives of General Psychiatry*, **51**, 294–301.

Susser, M.

1987   *Epidemiology, health, and society: Selected papers.* New York: Oxford University Press.

Swartz, L.

1985a   Anorexia nervosa as a culture-bound syndrome. *Social Science and Medicine*, **20**, 725–730.

1985b   Issues for cross-cultural psychiatric research in South Africa. *Culture, Medicine and Psychiatry*, **9**, 59–74.

1986   Transcultural psychiatry in South Africa. Part I. *Transcultural Psychiatric Research Review*, **23**, 273–303.

1987a   Illness negotiation: The case of eating disorders. *Social Science and Medicine,* **24,** 613–618.

1987b   Transcultural psychiatry in South Africa. Part II. *Transcultural Psychiatric Research Review,* **24,** 5–30.

1988   Some comments on the draft ethical code for clinical psychologists. *South African Journal of Psychology,* **18,** 17–20.

1989   *Aspects of culture in South African psychiatry.* Unpublished Ph.D. dissertation, University of Cape Town.

1991a   The politics of Black patients' identity: Ward-rounds on the 'Black side' of a South African psychiatric hospital. *Culture, Medicine and Psychiatry,* **15,** 217–244.

1991b   The reproduction of racism in South African mental health care. *South African Journal of Psychology,* **21,** 240–246.

1992   On the edge: Ward-rounds in a South African psychiatric casualty unit. *Social Science and Medicine,* **35,** 1115–1122.

1995   The politics of culture and mental illness: The case of South Africa. In I. Al-Issa (Ed.). *Handbook of culture and mental illness: An international perspective* (pp. 73–91). Madison: International Universities Press.

1996   Culture and mental health in the rainbow nation: Transcultural psychiatry in a changing South Africa. *Transcultural Psychiatric Research Review,* **33,** 119–136.

Swartz, L., Ben-Arie, O., & Teggin, A. F.
1985   Subcultural delusions and hallucinations: Comments on the Present State Examination in a multi-cultural context. *British Journal of Psychiatry,* **146,** 391–394.

Swartz, L., Drennan, G., & Crawford, A.
1997   Changing language policy in mental health services: A matter of interpretation? In D. Foster, M. Freeman., & Y. Pillay (Eds.). *Mental health policy issues for South Africa* (pp. 166–180). Cape Town: MASA Multimedia.

Swartz, L., & Foster, D.
1984   Images of culture and mental illness: South African psychiatric approaches. *Social Dynamics,* **10,** 17–25.

Swartz, L., Gibson, K., & Swartz, S.
1990   State violence in South Africa and the development of a progressive psychology. In N. C. Manganyi & A. du Toit (Eds.). *Political violence and the struggle in South Africa* (pp. 234–264). London: Macmillan.

Swartz, L., & Levett, A.
1989   Political repression and children in South Africa: The social construction of damaging effects. *Social Science and Medicine,* **28,** 741–750.

Swartz, L., & Maw, A.

1996   Language accessibility and training in clinical psychology: Experiences at the UCT Child Guidance Clinic. Proceedings of *Communication for the health professions in a multi-lingual society* (Ed. W. Loening), Durban, July, pp. 68–82.

Swartz, L., & Miller, T.

1992a   *Final report: The epidemiology of psychological distress and disorder in Mamre (Grant 15/1/3/2/156).* Report for the Institute for Research Development of the Human Sciences Research Council, Pretoria.

1992b   Not 'women and stress': Negotiating a role for clinical psychologists in a South African community health project. Paper presented at the annual meeting of the American Anthropological Association, San Francisco, December 1992.

Swartz, L., & Sheward, D.

1995   The epidemiology of anorexia nervosa and bulimia nervosa in South Africa. *South African Journal of Continuing Medical Education*, **13**, 541–542.

Swartz, S.

1995   Colonizing the insane: Causes of insanity in the Cape, 1891 – 1920. *History of the Human Sciences*, **8**, 39–57.

1996   *Colonialism and the production of psychiatric knowledge in the Cape, 1891–1920.* Unpublished Ph.D. dissertation, University of Cape Town.

Swartz, S., Dowdall, T., & Swartz, L.

1986   Clinical psychology and the 1985 crisis in Cape Town. *Psychology in Society*, **5**, 131–138.

Swartz, S., & Swartz, L.

1987   Talk about talk: Metacommentary and context in the analysis of psychotic discourse. *Culture, Medicine and Psychiatry*, **11**, 395–416.

Swift, J.

1965/1726 *Gulliver's travels*. London: Methuen.

Szasz, T.

1961   *The myth of mental illness*. New York: Hoeber and Harper.

1971   *The manufacture of madness*. London: Routledge and Kegan Paul.

Tau, J.

1989   Family therapy: Is it relevant to the experience of South Africa's third world communities? In J. B. Mason & J. Rubenstein (Eds.). *Family therapy in South Africa today* (pp. 37–39). Congella, South Africa: South African Institute of Marital and Family Therapy.

The Lancet

1977   Apartheid and mental health care (Editorial). *The Lancet*, **2**, 491.

Thom, R. G. M., Zwi, R. M., & Reinach, S. G.

1993   The prevalence of psychiatric disorder in a primary care clinic in Soweto. *South African Medical Journal*, **83**, 653–655.

Thornton, R.

1988   Culture: A contemporary definition. In E. Boonzaier & J. Sharp (Eds.). *South African keywords: The use and abuse of political concepts* (pp. 1–16). Cape Town: David Philip.

Thorpe, M. S.

1982   *Psycho-diagnostics in a Xhosa Zionist Church.* Unpublished M.A. thesis, Rhodes University, Grahamstown.

Tillman, J. G., Nash, M. R., & Lerner, P. M.

1994   Does trauma cause dissociative pathology? In S.J. Lynn & W. Rhue (Eds.). *Dissociation: Clinical and theoretical perspectives* (pp. 395–414). New York: Guilford Press.

Toulmin, S.

1978   Psychic health, mental clarity, self-knowledge and other virtues. In H.T. Engelhardt, Jr. & S.F. Spicker (Eds.). *Mental health: Philosophical perspectives* (pp. 55–70). Dordrecht: Reidel.

True, W. R.

1990   Epidemiology and medical anthropology. In T. M. Johnson & C. F. Sargent (Eds.). *Medical anthropology: Contemporary theory and method* (pp. 298–318). New York: Praeger.

Turkle, S.

1995   *Life on the screen: Identity in the age of the Internet.* London: Phoenix.

Turner, T. J.

1994   Bodies and anti-bodies: Flesh and fetish in contemporary social theory. In T. J. Csordas (Ed.). *Embodiment and experience: The existential ground of culture and self* (pp. 27–47). Cambridge: Cambridge University Press.

Turner, V.

1968   *The drums of affliction.* Oxford: Clarendon.

1969   *The ritual process: Structure and anti-structure.* London: Routledge & Kegan Paul.

Turton, R. W.

1986   *Stressful life events and illness among urban blacks.* Unpublished M.A. thesis, University of Witwatersrand, Johannesburg.

Turton, R. W., & Chalmers, B. E.

1990   Apartheid, stress and illness: The demographic context of distress reported by African South Africans. *Social Science and Medicine*, **31**, 1191–1200.

Tyrer, P.
1982   Anxiety states. In E. S. Paykel (Ed.). *Handbook of affective disorder* (pp. 59–69). Edinburgh: Churchill Livingstone.

Van der Geest, S., & Whyte, S. R. (Eds.)
1988   *The context of medicines in developing countries.* Dordrecht: Kluwer.

Van der Spuy, H. I. J., & Shamley, D. A. F. (Eds.)
1978   *The psychology of apartheid: A psychosocial perspective on South Africa.* Washington, D.C.: University Press of America.

Van Os, J., Castle, D. J., Takei, N., Der, G., & Murray, R. M.
1996   Psychotic illness in ethnic minorities: Clarification from the 1991 census. *Psychological Medicine,* **26**, 203–208.

Vasquez, C., & Javier, R. A.
1991   The problem with interpreters: Communicating with Spanish-speaking patients. *Hospital and Community Psychiatry,* **42**, 163–165.

Vaughn, C. E., & Leff, J. P.
1976   The influence of family and social factors on the course of psychiatric illness: A comparison of schizophrenic and depressed neurotic patients. *British Journal of Psychiatry,* **129**, 125–137.

Vaughn, C. E., Snyder, K. S., Jones, S., Freeman, W. B., & Falloon, I. R. H.
1984   Family factors in schizophrenic relapse: A California replication of the British research on expressed emotion. *Archives of General Psychiatry,* **129**, 125–137.

Velimirovic, B.
1990   Is integration of traditional and western medicine really possible? In J. Coreil & J. D. Mull (Eds.). *Anthropology and primary health care* (pp. 51–78). Boulder, Colorado: Westview Press.

Vogelman, L.
1986   Apartheid and mental health. Proceedings of the Organization for Appropriate Social Services in Southern Africa 'Apartheid and Mental Health' Conference (pp. 3–12). Johannesburg: OASSSA.

Walt, G. (Ed.)
1990   *Community health workers in national programmes.* Milton Keynes: Open University Press.

Warner, R.
1985   *Recovery from schizophrenia: Psychiatry and political economy.* London. Routledge and Kegan Paul.
1992   Comment on Cohen, Prognosis for schizophrenia in the Third World. *Culture, Medicine and Psychiatry,* **16**, 85–88.
1994   *Recovery from schizophrenia: Psychiatry and political economy* (2nd ed.). London: Routledge.

Waxler, N. E.

1977   Is mental illness cured in traditional societies? A theoretical analysis. *Culture, Medicine and Psychiatry*, **1**, 233–253.

1979   Is outcome for schizophrenia better in nonindustrial societies? The case of Sri Lanka. *Journal of Nervous and Mental Diseases*, **167**, 144–158.

Waxler-Morrison, N.

1992   Comment on Cohen, Prognosis for schizophrenia in the Third World. *Culture, Medicine and Psychiatry*, **16**, 77–80.

Webster's new twentieth century dictionary of the English language (2nd edition)

1978   Revised by editorial staff under the general supervision of Jean L McKechnie. USA (city not stated): William Collins & World Publishing.

Weedon, C.

1987   *Feminist practice and poststructuralist theory*. Oxford: Basil Blackwell.

Weiss, M.

1997   Explanatory model interview catalogue (EMIC): Framework for comparative study of illness. *Transcultural Psychiatry*, **34**, 235–263.

Wessely, S.

1990   Old wine in new bottles: Neurasthenia and 'ME'. *Psychological Medicine*, **20**, 35–53.

West, L. J., & Martin, P. R.

1994   Pseudo-identity and the treatment of personality change in victims of captivity and cults. In S. J. Lynn & J. W. Rhue (Eds.). *Dissociation: Clinical and theoretical perspectives* (pp. 268–288). New York: Guilford Press.

West, M. E.

1975   *Bishops and prophets in a Black city: African independent churches in Soweto, Johannesburg*. Cape Town: David Philip, and London: Rex Collings.

White, G. M.

1982   Cultural knowledge of 'mental disorder'. In A. J. Marsella & G. M. White (Eds.). *Cultural conceptions of mental health and therapy* (pp. 69–95). Dordrecht: Reidel.

Wig, N. N., Menon, D. K., Bedi, H., Ghosh, A., Kuipers, L., Leff, J., Korten, A., Day, R., Sartorius, N., Ernberg, G., & Jablensky, A.

1987   Expressed Emotion and schizophrenia in North India. I. Cross-cultural transfer of ratings of relatives' Expressed Emotion. *British Journal of Psychiatry*, **151**, 156–160.

Wig, N. N., Menon, D. K., Leff, J., Kuipers, L., Ghosh, A., Day, R., Korten, A., Ernberg, G., Sartorius, N., Jablensky, A., Nielsen, J. A., & Thestrup, G.

1987   Expressed Emotion and schizophrenia in North India. II. Distribution of Expressed Emotion components among relatives of schizophrenic patients in Aarhus and Chandigarh. *British Journal of Psychiatry*, **151**, 161–165.

Williams, P., & Bellantuono, C.
1991   Long-term tranquilliser use: The contribution of epidemiology. In J. Gabe
        (Ed.). *Understanding tranquilliser use: The role of the social sciences* (pp. 69–91).
        London: Tavistock/ Routledge.

Wing, J. K.
1978   *Reasoning about madness*. Oxford: Oxford University Press.
1983   Use and misuse of PSE. *British Journal of Psychiatry*, **143**, 111–117.

Wing, J. K., Bebbington, P., & Robins, L. N. (Eds.)
1981   *What is a case? The problem of definition in psychiatric community surveys*.
        London: Grant McIntryre.

Wing, J. K., Cooper, J. E., & Sartorius, N.
1974   *The measurement and classification of psychiatric symptoms: An instruction
        manual for the PSE and Catego Program*. London: Cambridge University Press.

Wood, C. S.
1990   Maori community health workers: A mixed reception in New Zealand.
        In J. Coreil & J. D. Mull (Eds.). *Anthropology and primary health care*
        (pp. 123–136). Boulder, Colorado: Westview Press.

World Bank
1993   *World Bank development report 1993: Investing in health*. New York: Oxford
        University Press.

World Health Organization (WHO)
1973   *The international pilot study of schizophrenia*. Geneva: WHO.
1977   *Apartheid and mental health care: A preliminary review*. Publication MNH/77.5.
        Geneva: World Health Organization.
1978   Primary health care: Report of the international conference on primary
        health care. Alma Ata, USSR, 6–12 September. Jointly sponsored by the
        WHO and UNICEF. Geneva: World Health Organization.
1979   *Schizophrenia. An international follow-up study*. Chichester: John Wiley
        and Sons.
1992   *ICD–10 classification of mental and behavioural disorders (ICD-10)*. Geneva:
        World Health Organization.

Wurtzel, E.
1994   *Prozac nation*. Boston: Houghton Mifflin.

Yach, D., Matthews, K., & Buch, E.
1990   Urbanisation and health: Methodological difficulties in undertaking
        epidemiological research in developing countries. *Social Science and
        Medicine*, **31**, 507–514.

Young, A.
1980   The discourse on stress and the reproduction of conventional knowledge.
        Social Science and Medicine, **14B**, 133–146.

1995   *The harmony of illusions: Inventing posttraumatic stress disorder.* Princeton,
        New Jersey: Princeton University Press.

Zuckerman, B., & Brown, E. R.
1993   Maternal substance abuse and infant development. In C. H. Zeanah, Jr.
        (Ed.). *Handbook of infant mental health* (pp. 143–158). New York:
        Guilford Press.

Zwi, A., Marks, S., & Andersson, N.
1988   Introduction. Health, apartheid and the Frontline States. *Social Science and
        Medicine, 27,* 661–666.

Author index

Subject index